John's Story: Through the Valley and Beyond
Copyright @ 2007 by Sara Jane White. All rights reserved.

Registration Number: TXu-1-576-630

Published by
Sara Jane White
718 Montclair Blvd.
Sugar Land, TX 77478

First Printing, June 2007
ISBN: 978-0-9796484-0-3

This book is printed on acid-free paper.
Manufactured in the United States of America

JOHN'S STORY: THROUGH THE VALLEY AND BEYOND

By Sara Jane White

*In Memory of
John Warren, 1961-2004*

and

*Dedicated to
Lisa, Mary Kaitlin and Carly*

Forward

I first met John Warren in San Antonio in 1978 at the wedding of John's mother Sara Jane White and my friend and colleague Bob White. At Bob's daughter's wedding festivities in 2001, I got to know John a bit more. Vivid in my memory is John's dry but keen sense of humor. But most of all, I can picture his tender attentiveness toward Lisa and his two young daughters Carly and Mary Kaitlin.

In 2003, I heard about the second invasion of brain cancer into John's body. From the moment of my friend Bob's e-mail, I began daily prayer for John, his doctors, Lisa, Carly, Mary Kaitlin, and Bob and Sara Jane. My old childhood friend Colonel Larry Messner and his Lutheran congregation in North Conway, New Hampshire joined in weekly prayer for John, his family and his doctors. We knew about his medical miracle of a cure for the brain cancer twenty years before. Our prayers were filled with hope for a second miracle for John.

The second miracle unfortunately was not a lengthy extension of John's life, but the amazing, courageous and inspiring way that John faced his brain cancer. John assertively cooperated with his doctors in his treatment decisions and processes.

John's loving and remarkably resourceful mother has recorded **JOHN'S STORY** in a clear, inspiring and poignant way. Her account captures many inspiring and instructive dimensions of **JOHN'S STORY** for everyone who reads it.

Sara Jane chose to provide the details of John's **illness, diagnosis and treatments** in the doctors' own words as they are found in medical records. She also describes in important ways how John interacted with and tested his doctors. John in his own steady, low-key way inspired his doctors and other patients whose lives he touched. One detail that Sara Jane provides that captured and condensed the essence of this point for me is her description of John's "Moses Stick" and its meaning.

The ways in which John, Lisa, his mother Sara Jane and other members of his devoted family participated in John's treatment can provide inspiration and solid role modeling for brain cancer patients' families.

The **clergy and prayer-offering congregations** that joined in John's battle against brain cancer are carefully described. They can provide for guidance, inspiration and instruction for readers about how helpful well-attuned pastors and churches can be to patients who face brain cancer.

John's **employer and coworkers** demonstrate touching and inspiring evidence of what the very best in loyalty is for employers and employees. Sara Jane's descriptions of the gentle humor and good will gestures of these kind folks brought tears to my eyes. We seldom see such loyalty and compassion in our modern world of the 'bottom line worshippers'.

We learn in Sara Jane's account about John's guitar and the comfort music brought to John's life. Sara Jane shares with us readers the poems John wrote about his beloved grandfather and even one about his brain cancer! These poems are profound and convey the **special memorable music of John's soul**.

The exchange of letters, notes and **final earthly communications of John and his loved ones** that Sara Jane records reflects the special love that John and his "Angel" Lisa and their families have. That kind of Love walks beyond 'the valley of the shadow of Death'.

By Peter A. Olsson MD
Assistant Professor of Psychiatry, Dartmouth Medical School, Hanover, New Hampshire and Adjunct Clinical Professor of Psychiatry at Baylor College of Medicine, Houston.

CHAPTER 1

ENTERING THE VALLEY

"Until now, I did not know how much I was loved."

The phone rang on a Saturday afternoon, July 9, 1983. When Bob answered, it was John calling from College Station where he was attending summer school at Texas A&M University. He said that he was sick and that he was coming home this evening so that Mother could take care of him. I was away when the call came in. When I returned home, Bob met me at the door with the news. We both knew that John had to be really sick to seek help, as he was quite independent and would take care of himself if at all possible. We anxiously calculated from the approximate time of his call when he would arrive at our home, which is about a 90 mile drive from College Station. We estimated his arrival time between 6 and 7 in the evening, depending upon the exact time that he left College Station. But 6, 7 and 8 PM came and went, and John was not home yet.

We could not get in touch with him. We had no cell phones in 1983, and he had no line phone where he was staying. He was spending the summer in a small house trailer that he had purchased with money he had saved from previous jobs. He had stayed in it for several months the year before, while working in a West Texas oil field after taking a semester off during the second half of his sophomore year at the University of Texas. He had gone to the West Texas oil fields partly for the adventure and partly to be near his steady girlfriend, Susan. He and Susan met and started dating while they were both attending UT. Then Susan decided to transfer to Sul Ross College in Alpine, Texas, near the Big Bend National Park and closer to her father's ranch in New Mexico. Together they decided that John would go to West Texas as well, where he would work in the oil fields as a "rough neck." During her one semester as a student there, she and John continued dating. At the end of the spring semester, they both decided to leave West Texas and enter Texas A&M University in the fall as juniors. Upon entering A&M, John changed his major from accounting to petroleum engineering. He thought this was definitely a better fit for him, since he was a young man who loved the out-of-doors and dreaded the thought of a full time desk job. During his first year at A&M, he rented fairly typical off-campus student housing, but for summer school he decided to live in his little trailer in a trailer park near campus. John had started taking summer courses in order to make up for having been off a semester and changing universities as well as his major. With two semesters of summer school before the fall semester, John hoped to be able to receive his diploma the following summer of 1984.

Now, Bob and I were getting more and more anxious with the hours passing without John's arrival home. We talked by phone to the manager of the trailer park. They had no firm information as to when John left, though they checked and found that he was no longer there. As the hours wore on and we became more concerned, I called the highway patrol to find out if any accidents had been reported on the highway between College Station and Sugar Land. None had, but they would put out an alert for John's car. For his 22nd birthday on June 3, I had given him a new bright red car, a small American Motors "hatch back." He had had the car for only about 5 weeks. At least I assumed, he would not have car trouble. We anxiously continued our waiting.

At about midnight, John came in. He was very pale, had lost weight and was very obviously sick, with a noticeable sag on the left side of his face. But he was alive and he was home, where he needed to be so that we could nurse him back to health. We rejoiced in what I now call the "first miracle," which was that he somehow made it home. After grateful hugs and sighs of relief, he told us that he had been too sick to leave right after he called home. He had to wait several more hours for the vomiting and headache to subside. It was then that he managed to get out of the bed, slip into sandals, a pair of jeans and a shirt, and then get his black Labrador *Beaux* (pronounced *Bo*) into the car with him. (John's canine companion was given his name with the elaborate spelling by his proud new owner six years before when he was 16.) Now the two of them started the 90 mile drive home. But unfortunately, even more delay followed.

Barely beyond the city limits of College Station, John's new car had a blow out. To make matters worse, it happened in front of a training facility for police dogs. With John and *Beaux* parked on the side of the road at the edge of the kennels, the police dogs became very agitated. At that point, John warned *Beaux* in no uncertain terms that he had better behave, because if he escaped from the car, he was on his own! Then John went to work to the sound of a chorus of angry dogs, barking and growling from the confines of their kennels with *Beaux* answering in kind. John somehow managed to get the standard size tire off and put the small spare on his car, while coping not only with the distraction of the dogs, but also with double vision, a headache, and a bed of red ants near where he had to put his feet down. Fortunately *Beaux* heeded his warning and stayed safely inside the car while he finished changing the tire. Then John and *Beaux* once again started the arduous drive home. John drove very slowly and carefully for the nearly 90 miles remaining. He faced the long dark and lonely road hoping that the small supposedly "temporary" spare tire would hold up and coping with his weakened physical condition and vision problems as best he could. It took a survivor's spirit not to give up. John was to prove over and over again that he had an indomitable spirit and great courage. This was only the beginning.

After finally getting home, John sipped a little warm soup and then went to bed – exhausted and still complaining of a headache. Other symptoms were abated for the time being. I told John before he went to sleep, that we would go to the emergency room in the morning unless he was remarkably better. The next morning, Sunday, he was not better and so we went directly to the emergency room at MacGregor Clinic.

I had recently changed my health insurance to a new Health Maintenance Organization, Pru Care. John had just turned 22 and since he was still a full-time college student, he was eligible for coverage which I had continued for him. MacGregor Clinic was the Houston clinic that served the Pru Care Health Maintenance Organization. I had little experience with Pru Care or any HMO until then, either positive or negative, as I had only changed my private health insurance a few short months before John's diagnosis. My inexperience with the workings of an HMO would change quickly.

The Pru Care emergency room doctor that examined John did not attempt to diagnose his problem. He did prescribe a strong pain killer for the headache and sent us home with instructions to take him to see a physician at MacGregor Clinic the next day, if he did not improve. At the crack of dawn on Monday, I was on the phone trying to make an appointment with an internist (primary physician) at MacGregor Clinic as his condition had not improved very much if any. The receptionist insisted that John could not be seen that day. I told her that the emergency room doctor's records should be available, referring John for an appointment this morning. I insisted that this was an emergency, but I continued to meet with resistance to the point that I felt the need to sound as threatening as I could. My way of doing that was to say that either they work John in this morning or I would take him to the Emergency Room of the hospital where my doctor husband hospitalized patients. I was sure that the other hospital would see John. My last words on the subject were "I will deal with you later." To my satisfaction this approach made an impact, and I was soon asked if we could be there in 40 minutes.

It was a good 40 minute drive to the clinic from our home and at the time I got the appointment, John was still in bed. Yet I assured her that we would be there in 40 minutes. John, in bed and so very sick when told of the appointment, hastily got up and slipped on his jeans and a T-shirt that he had worn home on Saturday night. We made it to the appointment on time. From that time forward, excellent medical care was received at every juncture from John's diagnosis to presurgery, surgery and subsequent treatment. I heard from others along the way that this new HMO was excellent at mobilizing resources for very sick patients. Patients with ordinary health maintenance problems were more likely to have complaints about the HMO's health care delivery on a day to day basis. However, I stayed with the system until it folded nearly 20 years later, and I always had confidence and satisfaction in the health care that John and I received, emergency or otherwise. I do not think that overall, it had any thing to do with Bob being a doctor as I never mentioned it again.

When we arrived at the clinic on Monday morning, July 11, we were quickly taken to see an internist, Dr. Harroun, who examined John and took a medical history which included the following notations.

> *John had had persistent bifrontal headaches for about 3-4 weeks. They would occur most severely in the morning and then get somewhat better throughout the day. He began to notice blurred vision and 7-9 days before admission he began to also have episodic nausea with vomiting. His gait became somewhat unstable and this prompted him to come to the clinic* (where he saw Dr. Harroun). The report also noted that his medical history was *unremarkable. He doesn't smoke cigarettes. He drinks beer usually on the weekends, and is a student at Texas A&M where he is a senior engineering student.*

In his next paragraph, Dr. Harroun revealed another aspect of his medical history that we had shared with him that was more troubling. It stated as follows:

> *Significantly, 6 or 7 years ago he had what sounds like visual scotomata and was evaluated in San Antonio with a CT scan. He was reassured about this condition which did not recur. Nevertheless, it prevented him from being insured at an inexpensive rate.*

Based upon a recalled conversation between John's father and Dr. Joel Y. Rutman, recorded in a 1980 letter for insurance purposes, John's condition was characterized as *cerebral artery ischemia*. Dr. Rutman was the physician who treated John at the Santa Rosa Children's Hospital in San Antonio when he was 15 years old for symptoms that appeared to be transient and brought on by exertion while lifting weights. I remembered the diagnosis as an "atypical migraine." In any event, the doctors involved did not seem to really know what was going on, as there was nothing apparent from the imaging technology available at the time (1976).

After taking his medical history and conducting a physical examination, Dr. Harroun ordered John's immediate admission to the Medical Center Del Oro Hospital, which was right across the street from the McGregor Clinic on Greenbrier in Houston. This relatively small hospital was at the edge of the Houston Medical Center area, where the M.D. Anderson Cancer Treatment Center and other highly regarded medical institutions, such as Baylor College of Medicine, are located.

According to the admission slip that John and I took across the street to the hospital, Dr. Harroun suspected spinal meningitis. Therefore John was taken immediately to a private room in the isolation unit of the hospital. The usual procedures for entry were waived in order to get him quickly into his room and away from others. We were there for most of the day apprehensively waiting together except for the time when John was rolled away for x-rays and a CT scan.

We kept expecting someone to come to take him away again, this time for a spinal tap which a doctor had indicated earlier that they would do. But no one came as the afternoon wore on. I was beginning to feel irritation that staff had not come to take him for the spinal tap. Then, late in the day, three doctors entered his room. I immediately could tell by the number of doctors and the somber looks on their faces that something was very wrong. We soon found out to our horror that they had not taken John for a spinal tap because the pictures taken earlier in the day revealed a large mass in the right frontal lobe of his brain. Apparently, a spinal tap, given the pressure caused by the mass in his head, would have been fatal. Their explanation to us was frightening, but given in terms that we could understand. The doctors referred to the size of the mass as "large as a peach." The report filed by John Coan, M.D. that day, July 12, 1983, explained John's medical condition in more technical but perhaps even more frightening terms.

> *BILATERAL CAROTID ANGIOGRAPHY*
> *Diagnosis: Large right frontal mass, most compatible with a neoplasm.*
> *Comment: Injection of the right common carotid artery reveals a large (6 cms. by 4 1/2 cms.) mass in the right frontal region that shows moderate tumor staining in the early angiographic phase. There are abnormal tumor vessels within and about the periphery of the mass. Some early venous drainage is also appreciated. A large shift of the right anterior communicating artery from the right to left is appreciated and is in keeping with the size of this frontal lobe lesion. One or two small middle meningeal branches pass over the lesion on the right sided injection, but I am doubtful as to whether they actually supply the mass. Most of the circulation is believed to be derived*

from the internal carotid artery on the right side. The features of the lesion are most in keeping with a high-grade astrocytoma. Other differential possibilities such as a metastatic lesion or intra cerebral meningioma are believed to be less likely. In addition to the above findings, there is some compression and downward displacement of several of the ascending frontal arteries on the right side. Secondary to the mass effect.

On the injection of the left common carotid artery, the only noted change of significance is a shift of the left anterior cerebral artery from right to left by the mass effect in the opposite hemisphere.

John and I were both stunned. Still in a state of shock, we were given the names of three local neurosurgeons that were all available to Pru Care patients as needed. There were no neurosurgeons that were "in-house" at Macgregor Clinic, but fortunately they had top Houston neurosurgeons on call. I immediately called Bob. After he absorbed the shocking news, he told me that he knew two out of the three surgeons who by reputation were among the best in Houston. He suggested that we choose Dr. Richard Moiel, which we did, and he was called in on the case immediately.

Dr. Moiel started steroids that evening and explained to us that John would be on steroids for several days prior to surgery in order to get the swelling down sufficiently to do the craniotomy. John was kept in the hospital, taking steroids and other prescribed medication for pain for three nights prior to surgery. The surgery was scheduled for Thursday, July 14. During that time, I stayed with John constantly in his room. We talked, called friends and family, prayed, read the Bible, received visitors and hoped. His grandmother "Sancy," father Blair, step mother Charlotte and brother West came from San Antonio and his sister Sally and brother-in-law Jeff came from Chicago to John's bedside prior to the surgery. Friends and fellow employees from my workplace, the City of Bellaire, came to see John and some sent flowers to brighten his room during those three dreadful days of waiting.

During the time before surgery, Dr. Moiel visited John several times and in private, prepared me for the worst. He could not know for sure, but he thought that the mass in John's brain was a fast growing, malignant tumor. In relation to whether or not it was fast growing, he told us that he did not know what to hope for. He said that some times the fast growing tumors were more "confused" and thus could be more responsive to treatment.

I remember the night before surgery so well. The nurse brought me a bottle of special medicinal shampoo. She instructed me to wash and rinse John's hair thoroughly with it in three applications. I did this, praying that I was getting his thick hair clean enough to prevent infection. I also made a mental picture in my heart and soul of how he looked that night. He was calm and no longer in pain. Just to look at him or visit with him, you would not know that anything was wrong. And yet I knew that the surgery was very high risk and assuming that he survived it, his life and my life would probably never be the same again. When the day of surgery came, John's father Blair and stepmother Charlotte, his sister Sally (five years older than John) and brother West (four years older than John), and my mother (his grandmother "Sancy") and Bob were all there with me in the waiting room to anxiously await the outcome. It was a long and arduous wait with only sketchy information forthcoming until the surgery was over.

Soon after John was taken from surgery to the recovery area, Dr. Moiel rushed out to tell us very bad news. He had removed a large cancerous glioma brain tumor, he thought Grade IV. He could not get it all, and an emergency had developed. He now sought my permission to take John back into surgery to try to save his life. As he explained this to us, he had tears in his eyes and showed great compassion for John and his family. He told us that he had a daughter at A&M about John's age at the time. Of course, I quickly told him that I and all of us wanted him to go back to do everything that he could to save John's life. Soon, we saw John on a gurney speeding by us with three attendants at his side. They were taking him for another CAT scan, before returning him to the surgical suite for his second surgery of the day. This time it was not to remove the tumor but to try to save his life by relieving the pressure that had developed on his brain. I fell from my chair to my knees and prayed for his life as our family and friends stood by helplessly.

When Dr. Moiel came back to tell us about the second surgery, he said that John was doing much better. The good news was that he had not only succeeded in relieving the pressure, but in going back in, he had also been able to see better the remaining gross tumor and thus was able to remove it safely. Here is the report of the second surgery, as filed by Dr. Moiel.

> *Under satisfactory general endotracheal anesthesia after an emergency CAT scan was done, the patient clinically had hypertension and it appeared as though the residual mass was not only edema but some hematoma and tumor and the patient was immediately taken back to the Operating Room. His craniotomy flap was reopened and dissection carried down to the bone flap which was snapped free. He had a minimal epidural collection of blood. The dura was opened and the tumor cavity had within it some residual blood mostly superiorly where as some residual tumor was left. This was evacuated and the cranial tension relieved and the residual tumor that we could see along the cortical surface removed. Bipolar coagulation was used for hemostasis, bone wax on bone, some gelfoam pledgets. We waited a long period of time and the bleeding eventually ceased. Peroxide was used for irrigation. The dura was then loosely approximated and gelfoam placed over the surface of that. When the hemostasis was satisfactory the bone flap was replaced loosely with Vicryl suture and the scalp was closed as started. Two drains were used, one epidural and one sublaleal. Sterile dressing was applied. Supplemental Mannitol and steroids had been given. The patient was taken to the Recovery Room and Intensive Care in satisfactory condition.*

And so John's miracles were unfolding. Had there not been the hypertensive crises, there would not have been the second surgery, where Dr. Moiel could see and remove the residual tumor that he was unable to see and remove during the first surgery. In retrospect, after the fact that John survived the two brain surgeries in one day, I think that the most critical medical factor in John's remarkable long term recovery was getting the rest of the tumor that could be seen.

Nevertheless, we were told by Dr. Moiel and John's other doctors, that microscopic roots (tentacles) remained that would grow and spread rapidly, leaving little if any hope for long term survival.

After the two surgeries in one day, John remained in Intensive Care for three days. During that time, John's family went through great agony as we watched for progress in recovery from the surgery while learning more about his grave diagnosis. I was further traumatized by the thought of having to tell John that his tumor was cancerous. One of the ICU nurses reported to me soon after John was taken to ICU and regained consciousness that he had asked if it was cancer. He wanted to know. She was unhappy that he had not been told. But I had thought it best to hold back until he was a little stronger. Though John was awake the first evening in ICU, I thought that he was too weak and groggy to hear the bad news. It would be hard for any member of his family to face their 22 year old son, grandson, and brother with the awful news of the lethal malignancy that he was fighting, but the nurse was impatient. When I was leaving the hospital for a brief time to eat, she called me back from the car that I had just entered in order to urge me again to tell John. She explained to me that she was afraid John would not even live long enough to leave intensive care, and she thought that he needed to know his condition immediately in order to make last requests and tell his family good bye. She compared his cancer to the deadly "oat cell," which I had never heard of until then. This well intentioned nurse may have overstepped her boundaries in putting pressure on me to tell him before I was prepared to do so, but nevertheless she got my attention and in my fear and agony, I responded as best I knew how, but I did not tell him that night.

At the end of that tumultuous first day in ICU, I spent the night in a nearby hotel serving the medical center in order to stay near John and to return to the ICU waiting room early the next morning. Bob went home to sleep, get up early, see patients and then return to the hospital later in the day, but prior to that, he guided me to a restaurant for dinner. I was numb and felt completely lost. I did not know what to say and did not want to eat. I am sure that it was hard for Bob to find words of comfort, but somehow he did. Nevertheless, I remember that alone in the hotel room, with no one to hear me except perhaps a stranger in the next room, I cried until I fell to sleep.

The next morning, we had our first consultation with the MacGregor oncologist, Dr. Paul Gustafson, while standing outside the ICU where John was being cared for. I told him about the nurse's concerns and the difficulty I and other family members were having in being the one to tell John. He helped us by agreeing to tell John first. After Dr. Gustafson talked to John and gave him the bad news, I went in immediately to comfort and encourage him as best as I could. While I was there, I will never forget that John's body began trembling. Perhaps he was cold and traumatized or even suffered a mild convulsion. I leaned over his bed and held him close until the shaking stopped. Then I stayed with him for the rest of the strictly enforced visiting hour. That is what happened when John was told of his condition on the second day after the surgery.

During John's three days in ICU, Bob, being a doctor, had permission to put on "greens" and visit him at any time during the day or night. After his visits, he would report back to the rest of us, as we waited in the ICU waiting area between visiting hours. Fortunately, his reports documented John's continuing progress in recovering from the surgery. The rest of us would take turns going in one at a time to comfort and encourage him during the short periods when visits were allowed in ICU.

While John was still in ICU, Dr. Gustafson continued to make plans with us for his treatment. First of all, he gave us the pathologist report from the frozen section. His condition was diagnosed as Grade III rather than Grade 1V. Still a lethal glioma tumor, it was only slightly better news than the anticipated Grade IV and the recommended treatment was the same. He told us that in addition to radiation, they had a new protocol that he would like John to try. Without treatment, he did not think that John had more than six weeks to live. With treatment he was hoping that John's life could be extended, perhaps six months to a year or a little more. After this explanation, we all strongly agreed that Dr. Gustafson should proceed with the protocol for John. His consultation report that follows documents John's condition, our conversations with Dr. Gustafson, John's decision and supporting family consensus.

Date of consult: 7/15/83
Problem #1: *right frontal astrocytoma - status post-craniotomy, 7/14/83; grade 3 malignant astrocytoma.*

Subjective:
> *I was asked to see Mr. Warren in consultation. He was hospitalized on 7/11/83 for evaluation of persistent headache and the recent development of nausea and vomiting. For a 3-4 week period he had considerable bifrontal headache which would occur most severely in the morning and then get somewhat better throughout the day. He began to notice blurred vision and 7-9 days before admission began to also have episodic nausea with vomiting. His gait became somewhat unstable and this prompted him to come to the clinic where he saw Dr. Harroun and was felt to need hospital admission. His evaluation preoperatively consisted of an angiogram and a CT scan of the brain. CT showed a large right frontal mass which displaced structures from right to left. The possibility of early herniation was also noted. Angiogram revealed the large vascular mass which was supplied by the internal carotid artery on the right side. On 7/14/83 he was taken to the operating room where craniotomy was performed and a complete resection of the tumor was performed by Dr. Moiel. He is currently recuperating in the intensive Care Unit of Del Oro Hospital and has had an uncomplicated postoperative course thus far. ....*

Objective: Physical Examination
B/P 143/57; Pulse 98; Resp: 20 Temp: 99.2

> *He is alert, responsive, and answers all questions appropriately. His head is bandaged from the recent surgery. There is a very mild left facial weakness. The pupils are equally reactive to light and accommodation. Extra ocular movements are intact. Eye grounds are not examined.*
>
> *Bilateral grip strength is normal and symmetric. There is no evidence of weakness in the lower extremities.*
>
> *Chest and heart are normal. Abdomen is soft and non-tender. Legs are within normal limits. At this time, other than the mild left facial weakness, there is no evidence of neurologic dysfunction.*

Review of chart shows his electrolytes to be normal. His blood sugar is 215, his chemistries are completely normal. He is presently on hydrochlorothiazide 50 mg. p.o., b.i.d., Inderal 40 mg. p.o., b.i.d. and Nipride to control systolic hypertension. He is on Decadron 8 mg, q.i.d., Dilantin 100 mg., q 8 hours and Tagamet; 300 mg. Q 6 hours.

Pathology report on the tumor removed at the time of surgery reveals a malignant astrocytoma, Grade 3.

Assessment:

Malignant Astrocytoma status post-craniotomy with complete resection of tumor.

Recommendation:

I have spoken with both John and his family in regard to the seriousness of this medical problem. I have been quite frank with them in regard to the percentages involved and his chance for long term survival. I have recommended to them that we begin therapy this coming week with combined modality therapy consisting of radiotherapy, preceded by chemotherapy consisting of cis platinum and CCNU. I have contacted the radio-therapy department at Methodist Hospital and he is scheduled to be seen there on July 25, 1983 at 9:00 a.m. I anticipate that next week toward the end of the week prior to his discharge from Del Oro Hospital, we will administer chemotherapy consisting of the cis platinum at a dose of 200 mg given over one hour. He will then be started also on CCNU at a dose of 50 mg per meter square per day, which he will take during his first two days of radiotherapy. This will be given every 6 weeks. A second dose of the cis platinum will be given 4 weeks following the first. Prior to beginning his chemotherapy we will need to obtain a 24 hour urine for creatinine, protein and creatinine clearance.

Paul A. Gustafson, M.D.

Fortunately, there were no more crises for John while in ICU. On July 17, he was taken to a large, private suite at the end of the 7th floor of the hospital. There was a sofa bed and a round table and chairs in the room. I stayed with him day and night, sleeping on the sofa bed. One night I apparently was having a bad dream from the stress. John, in his self-effacing way, got out of his bed and came to wake me up and comfort me by telling me that he was "all right."

In the hospital and under the death sentence of an Astrocytoma III, his courage and grace emerged and remained his hallmark for the next 21 years. He found out during this time how many people loved him and supported him, including not only his family but also friends and hospital staff, not the least of which was Dr. Moiel. Several days after John was out of intensive care, he was strong enough to move around. At that point, Dr. Moiel asked if it would be OK with him and his family for the good doctor to wheel him down to radiology to show him pictures of the mass that he had removed from John's brain. John wanted to see the images, so with that, Dr. Moiel personally pushed his wheelchair to the area in the hospital where the X-rays could be viewed. On the way, John's father made an appreciative and complementary comment to Dr. Moiel, asking him how he or anyone could be a brain surgeon, to whom Dr. Moiel modestly replied; "Well, it beats pulling weeds."

John particularly bonded with an intensive care nurse named "LuLu." As John improved, another of the nurses on John's floor would come in when she was off-duty to play card games with him at the table in his large corner room. John's girlfriend, Susan, had gone to Spain to study Spanish for the summer. When she received word that John would have surgery to remove a mass from his brain, she cut short her stay in Spain, and flew home as soon as she could get a flight out. She could not get there before the surgery, but made it in time to visit him while he was still in the hospital. He was glad to see her, but I think that he probably knew already that their relationship could not continue in the face of his uncertain future. Her parents sent a huge flower arrangement to John, with a card in which they not only encouraged him to get well but referred to him in a lighted hearted way as a very handsome man! His Uncle Bob and long time friends from San Antonio and Alamo Heights High School drove over to see him, among them were his close friends, Cole Alexander, Rebbie Brem, Gary Boldt and Ashby McMullen. Ashby flew from Colorado where he was attending the Colorado School of Mines in order to be with John.

With his spirits lifted from all of the support he was receiving, John even asked me to bring his guitar to his hospital room, which he began to strum a little during his better moments as his strength was returning. Family, friends and even strangers continued to rally around him during the 12 days that he spent in the Del Oro Hospital. Word came to him of church groups and individuals praying for him around the United States and in places as far away as Nigeria. John was deeply touched by the love that was poured out. It was then that he found something very good in the catastrophe. He told me; "Until now, I never knew how much I was loved." Thus he began his spiritual recovery while still in the hospital, living each day to the fullest. This never changed.

His progress over his days in the hospital was steady and therefore Dr. Gustafson ordered his first cis platinum treatment to be given the day before his discharge on July 23. The procedure was considered a dangerous one. It involved running a catheter to his brain and slowly dripping the cis platinum into the cavity where the tumor had been removed. Medical Center Del Oro was reported to have had better success with this procedure than other hospitals in the Medical Center, because they had devised a filter to aid in preventing strokes, for which the patients were at risk. Once again, John was sent to a surgical suite, and once again, I waited anxiously for the outcome. John tolerated the treatment without complications. His second cisplatin treatment was scheduled for the first part of August. He would return to the hospital for an overnight stay, in order to be properly hydrated and monitored before and after the procedure. The day before he was to return for the second treatment, Hurricane Alicia paid Houston a visit, and the hospital had to reschedule. I was frightened about this delay, until Dr. Gustafson assured me that a week's delay would not be detrimental to the effectiveness of the treatment.

While John was still in the hospital, I had a call at home from law enforcement in College Station regarding a theft in the trailer park where John's little trailer was still parked. Letters to John were found in the trailer where the robbery had taken place, so John was a "suspect." I explained to the sheriff that John was in the hospital having had brain surgery, so he could not come to the phone. As it turned out, he was already in the hospital when the robbery occurred. Some vandals had broken into John's empty trailer and found the letters that Susan had written to John from Spain. They apparently took the letters and then spread them on the floor of the house trailer that they had entered to rob and vandalize. John had the "perfect" alibi. Not that he would have needed it in the long run, for the sheriff told me that trailer park owners and others that he questioned vouched for his character and emphasized what a nice and kind person that he was. He was always helping out when needed. Subsequently the sheriff found the culprits. After John was well enough to go with me, he and I retrieved his trailer from the park, and were much relieved to get it in a safer place until he could sell it.

    I remember driving John home on the day that he was released from the hospital. John was happy to be going home and I was happy too. However, it was scary for both of us for him to make the transition, leaving behind all of the special care and expertise provided at the hospital and given all of the uncertainty associated with his prognosis and further treatment. I suspect that I was more frightened, certainly more anxious, than John. On the way home, I drove rather slowly and very carefully, avoiding sudden stops that might jar him or worse still, throw him against the dashboard. In doing this, I made matters worse. As I slowly made my way on Highway 90, a traffic light changed. I reacted and stopped rather suddenly as the light was changing from yellow to red. A car of young people behind us slammed on their breaks, and then pulled up beside me. An angry young woman got out of the car on John's side, shaking her fist and cursing in a very threatening way. Our windows were rolled up, doors locked, and we did not respond. When the light changed, I gingerly drove away. I wondered if she would have behaved differently had she known our circumstances.

Chapter 2

RECOVERY

"Tie a knot and hang on."

John began radiation therapy as an outpatient of the Methodist Hospital on July 26. Under the protocol he should have received treatment five days per week for five weeks. He was to receive 4,500 rads to the whole brain and a "brain boost" of 1,080. It was very close to the maximum dose that they could give. For some reason, they mistakenly scheduled him for four days a week. On August 1, the mistake was discovered. He requested that the four day per week schedule be continued because of the need to register at the University of Houston for the 1983 fall semester. His overall dosage would be the same as it would have been had it been spread over five days per week. I was anxious about this slight deviation in his treatment protocol. But the doctors assured me that since he was tolerating the more concentrated dosage well, the change would not harm him because it would not change the ultimate dosage. Thus the request was granted.

John had wanted to return to Texas A & M in the fall, but Dr. Moiel and Dr. Gustafson believed that it was too soon for that. However, John was determined to resume work on his degree, so his doctors agreed with Plan B, which was to live at home and take courses at the University of Houston during the fall. During the fall semester, John worked hard at his studies. The work was made more difficult because of having difficulty hearing. Therefore, he had a hearing test, which proved there was some loss of hearing, though hearing aids were not recommended. John attributed the hearing loss to shot gun blasts from hunting as a boy. In retrospect, we now know that this is a common occurrence with the use of cis platinum.

His radiotherapy was completed on September 9. At that time, he had already been back in school for about two weeks of classes, taking nine hours of needed course work that would be transferable to A&M. For the first few weeks of the semester, due to the possible side effects of radiation, the doctors did not release him to drive, so I transported him to school and back home. On the day after the last day of radiation, John said that he was so relieved that the radiation therapy was complete. He confided that he was getting worried about his ability to continue tolerating the treatment while going to school. He described how it felt during the last few treatments, which was as though his brain was turning to a bowl of mush or jelly. Once the treatment stopped, he recovered from these troublesome side effects and successfully completed the nine hours of his University of Houston semester.

He would continue the CCNU that Dr. Gustafson had prescribed as part of the protocol until the next summer. Every six weeks he would take large doses as prescribed for two days. It would initially make him nauseated and he would vomit and lose his appetite. But after a few days, he would get better although the medicine would stay in his system until time for the next dose. He lost about 35 pounds, then weighing only about 140 pounds though he was 6'2." He lost his hair and long eye lashes. After radiation was completed, his thick and wavy dark brown hair eventually was replaced with thin fine hair that looked more like baby hair. He had never had adolescent acne, but the radiation caused skin problems, with dryness and acne. The skin problems cleared and his eye lashes grew back after radiation, but he did not even begin to regain his normal weight until after the year of chemotherapy was completed. John occasionally commented to me on the impact of his illness on his youthful appearance. With his hair gone, a large scar on his scalp, and his body thin and pale, he looked in the mirror one day when I was nearby and said "I'm ugly!" My heart hurt as I assured him wholeheartedly that that was not so. But I suggested that if he wanted to consider being fitted for a wig, the doctors had given me the thick dark hair that they had shaved from his head before the surgery. He firmly rejected this idea. Instead he said; "I will play with the cards I have been dealt." Therefore, he would be who he was, and now that included being a person fighting a brain tumor. Thus he continued his life with dignity and self respect and he did not look back.

He did not have previous friends and acquaintances at the University of Houston, or in our community, as he had grown up in

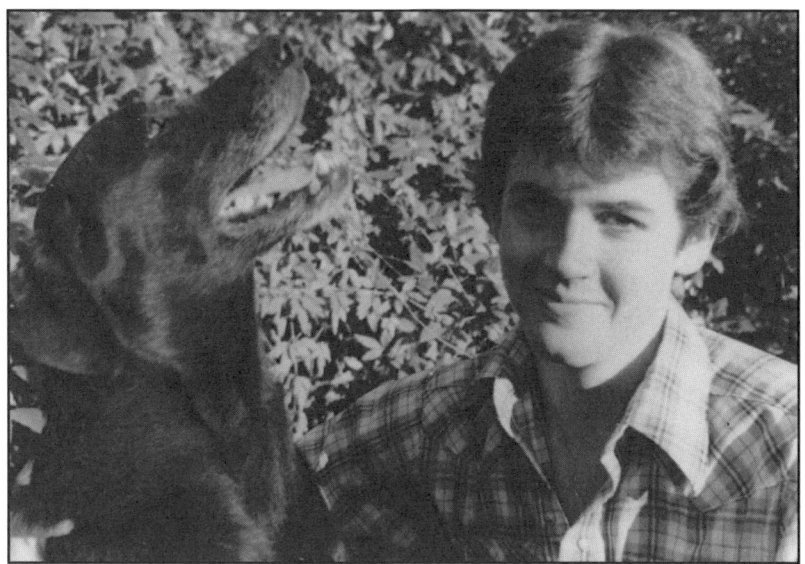
Girlfriend Susan took this photo of John and his dog "Beaux" before the brain tumor (1982)

San Antonio. Never before had he lived over an extended period of time in the Houston area. He was lonely, as it was hard to make new friends, while on chemotherapy and fighting a brain tumor. His energy was limited, and among strangers, he no longer "looked" the part of the "typical" young male college student. As I recall, he did make a new friend who was also transferring to A&M. In addition, he became pool playing friends with a young man from Ethiopia, attending the University of Houston and working as an intern part time in planning for the City of Bellaire, where I was City Planner. But for the most part, he spent his time outside of classes studying at home or in the library.

John and his girl friend Susan did not sustain their relationship under these difficult circumstances. He put aside the thought of dating anyone new, as he did not want to get involved in the foreseeable future, only to have a recurrence bring a new relationship to a sad and abrupt ending. With all of this, he may have been discouraged, but he was far from defeated.

Even before John left the hospital, his family was looking at possible ways to supplement his medical treatment that might help him. His sister Sally found a book on macrobiotic diets and cancer, written by a doctor who had gone on a macrobiotic diet in combination with his medical treatment when fighting colon cancer. As a result of reading that book, I bought several macrobiotic cookbooks and started cooking macrobiotic meals as soon as John was home from the hospital, but only after checking with our doctors, to make sure that they thought it would not be detrimental to the effectiveness of his medical treatment. John and I even took some macrobiotic cooking lessons at the East/West Center located in Houston's Montrose neighborhood. We learned how to cook with sea weed and all kinds of greens, almost an entirely vegetarian diet except for an occasional piece of fish. Miso soup was an important part of the diet. Miso had been found to greatly reduce the effects of radiation in Japan, when included in the diet of nurses and patients in hospitals following the atomic bombs of Hiroshima and Nagasaki. We were totally committed to the diet for six weeks. But then, John rebelled and asked for a good steak and some Mexican food. After that, we were much less rigid about the diet, continuing the miso soup and a lot of good vegetables, but adding more meat and fish than was recommended.

 Bob knew a psychologist who had gotten interested in *visioning* as a supplemental treatment modality for cancer patients. At our urging, John made an appointment with her. She taught him techniques of visioning. The idea was for the patient to imagine something that would attack the cancer cells, such as a "Pac Man" who would "gobble" up the unwanted cells. Since John, a seventh generation Texan, "naturally" loved to hunt with his friends and family, he chose a "gun" to "shoot" the cancer cells. After attending sessions with her for a month or more, John had a mystical experience in one session that he never forgot. He was visioning destroying the cancer cells by shooting them. An unsolicited "hand" appeared in his vision and took the gun from him. Then a "Voice" in the vision told John that from now on, do not worry, He would take care of it. Soon after that, John ended his trips to the therapist. He continued to follow his medical protocol, and went on with his life with a new sense of faith, hope and intimacy with God.

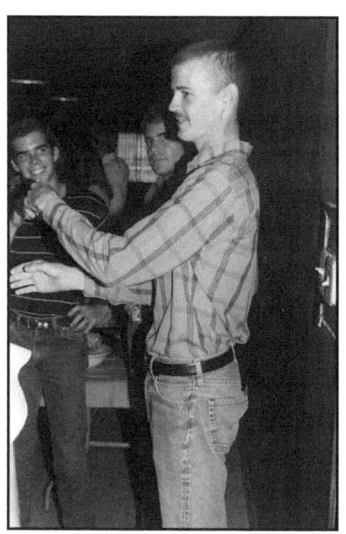
John's 23 birthday party

During his first year of chemotherapy and recovery, John did not have a recurrence to his doctor's relief and surprise. We were so thankful as each examination through the year would bring this good news. Still, all did not go smoothly. John developed a skull bone infection. At first he was given antibiotics, but they did not help. Then at Christmas time of 1983, he was put back in the hospital for a debridement of the bone in the infected area. I remember putting a little lighted tree with a music box in his room. He was there for several days before returning home on Christmas Eve. He then recuperated for the rest of the Christmas season at home. In January, he was well enough to start his first post tumor semester back at A&M. He was so glad to go back, though the work was more difficult for him now due to weakness from the chemotherapy and to difficulty he had in large classes hearing his professors well enough to keep up with the course work. Soon after returning to A&M, a new lesion appeared on his head which indicated to us that the bone infection might still be there. This was confirmed by his infectious disease doctor, and he returned home during spring break to reenter the hospital for a second debridement. He brought his books along to study but had few opportunities to open them, since the debridement caused terrible head aches while recovering. Nevertheless, he was determined to continue, so he returned to classes at the end of spring break and finished his semester, passing all of his courses.

At the end of his first year after the tumor was removed, we decided to have a big birthday party for John in a rented hall in San Antonio. His brother West engaged a musician named Darden Smith, who West chose because he especially liked his style of country and western singing and thought John would also, which he did. Thus we celebrated John's survival for one year after his cancer diagnosis with many friends and well wishers of all ages. John was still taking chemotherapy treatment (CCNU) and he was still way below his normal weight. But all things considered, he was doing very well because the tumor was still in remission. This made for a very good time at his big birthday celebration.

Shortly after his birthday, John reported to work for the Getty Oil Company at their Streetman Plant near Corsicana. This job was a requirement that he had to fulfill in order to receive his degree in Petroleum Engineering from Texas A&M. The University did not provide assistance in placing students in the required employment. He was helped by a kind friend of mine, who was a prominent civic leader in the City of Bellaire, a grandfatherly gentleman named Clyde Willbern. Clyde loved nothing better than giving a hand to young people. Mr. Willbern was a recently retired attorney for Getty Oil and thus was able to steer John toward this much needed job in the field of petroleum engineering.

When John arrived in Corsicana, he found a nice furnished garage apartment to rent. It was behind an attractive old Victorian house located on a shady lot across the street from the historic courthouse. Corsicana is the county seat of Navarro County. As is true of most courthouses of Texas, this 1905 brick and marble building is an awesome sight to behold. But John was there on a mission other than to see and enjoy Texas courthouses.

He was still taking the CCNU throughout those two and one half hot summer months that he lived and worked there. I was so worried about him, living alone and working under the conditions of being mostly out of doors or in a hot plant in the heat of a Texas summer, while his immune system was still under siege from chemotherapy. So I called a close friend Nancy Keeton, whose mother was from Corsicana. She still had relatives there, so I told her about John. She in turn, contacted her cousins. They invited John to their home for meals on several occasions. This was just about his only diversion, except for several trips that I made to see him, and a few trips he made to see family and friends in San Antonio and his sister in nearby Dallas.

John survived the summer and maintained his determination and optimism throughout his stay in Corsicana. Thus he completed the required field work for his degree program. But as the summer wore on, while still working at the job near Corsicana, a new and worrisome wound opened up on top of his head in a different location from the previous two lesions stemming from bone infection. Apparently the previous efforts had not stopped its spread.

Back in Houston, John's infectious disease doctor told him that plastic surgery would be required along with the third surgery in less than a year for bone debridement. That is, if we decided to treat it. John and I were not happy when the doctor said; "In a situation like this, it is hard to know what to do. We doctors must *do no harm*, and John's primary disease is not likely to stay in remission." But with positive input from John and me, he warily recommended proceeding with the surgery.

Samples of infected tissue analyzed from the previous two surgeries had not resulted in a specific finding as to the type of bacteria causing the infection. Therefore John had been treated only with broad spectrum antibiotics. This time, the pathologists were able to identify the bacteria specifically, a common type that causes acne. With this discovery, six weeks of intravenous antibiotics were prescribed that targeted the bacteria identified. The intravenous treatments were started before he left the hospital and then continued at home after his discharge. In the meantime, John completed his CCNU protocol at the end of August. As time went on, John admitted to me his frustration that the doctors took so long to find the offending common bacteria as they searched for a more exotic offender. In addition to the pain and suffering, the three surgeries had caused more scaring and disfigurement of his skull and hairline than would have been the case had the antibiotic been effective after one or even two surgeries.

Perhaps the saddest part of this third episode of bone infection for John was that just when he was expecting to return to A&M for the fall semester, free of chemotherapy, he was required to take off another semester in order to finish the intravenous antibiotics. John did not cry often, but the tears welled up in his beautiful brown eyes as he heard the news that it would not be feasible to go back to school yet. He tried to resist, but in the end, he realized that the importance of winning the fight against this infection rested on staying at home and receiving the IV's daily. Otherwise the bone infection would likely persist, invade the brain, and take his life.

During this difficult time, John's grandmother Sancy and her loyal friend and housekeeper of many years, Beatrice, came over to stay for several weeks with John. Bea and Sancy had been an important part of John's life, during the years we lived in San Antonio. As John grew up, they would see him often, and they helped me with baby sitting during those years when he was too young to stay home alone. Now, their visit was much appreciated, as I was gone during a large part of the day, back at my job as City Planner for the City of Bellaire. I needed to stay at work, since I had taken a six week leave of absence during the critical period of John's illness the previous summer. John enjoyed their company and I enjoyed knowing that they were there with him while I was away.

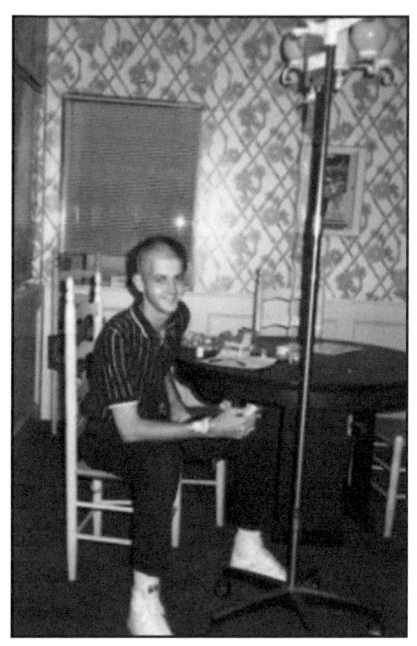

Missing a semester at TAMU for IV treatments.

Even with this new setback in meeting his goal of graduating from A&M, John kept his spirits up in many creative ways. One day between I V treatments, he drove into Houston to buy a cockatiel. He brought the bird home and named him *Maynard*. John tried very hard to turn him into a pet, and a talking one at that, but *Maynard* would have none of it. So John had to be content to feed him and to be amused by his cantankerous ways. John also read during this time, mostly western novels, which were always his favorites. John's dog *Beaux* remained his faithful companion during this trying time, when once again he had to postpone his pursuit of a Bachelors degree. In our concern for how difficult this time was for John, we even "relented" and let *Beaux* sleep in his bedroom! I also sold our ancient grand piano. It was in very bad condition, and needed to be completely rebuilt at a handsome price. For the price of its sale, I bought a rather plain new pool table which fit perfectly into our garden room. John played a lot of pool while stuck at home, and all of us enjoyed this diversion for years to come.

John's sister Sally had a couple of single girl friends, Danna and Liza, who lived in Dallas, where she and Jeff had recently moved after his graduation from Northwestern's Kellogg School of Business in Illinois. When these two young women heard from Sally of John's plight, they wrote to him. As he bided his time at home fighting the bone infection, he clearly enjoyed their attention as was reflected in his witty response to their letter.

> *Dear Friends of Sally, foxy and sweet:*
> *You sound like two that I would like to meet.*
> *I can't right now, but I'm not insane.*
> *My excuse is gross and involves some pain.*
> *So I won't see ya'all for a while,*
> *But I placed your letter in my file.*
> *The X's and O's sound great to me.*
> *Someday Dallas is where I'll be*
> *To meet you both, Danna and Liza*
> *And stuff our faces with beer and pizza!*
>   *XOXEROX ,*
>   *John*

While waiting to return to A&M, John tried his hand at writing more serious poetry as well. I love two of these poems that I saved through the years. (I would have saved them all, but John would tear up those he did not like before I salvaged them.) One that I managed to keep was called *Partners* and was written in memory of "Pop," his grandfather Westbrook, who had died suddenly just three years before in 1981 of a heart attack, while quail hunting in south Texas.

Pop and John had enjoyed many trips to the Cha Mar, a small ranch near San Antonio, that Pop and Sancy had bought for their retirement years. Before brother West and sister Sally went away to college, they too enjoyed trips to the Cha Mar. But John was younger and had more years to go there with Pop before time had to be given to higher education, young adult commitments and related responsibilities and pleasures. So Pop in his retirement and John in his boyhood would ride their horses, *Spangles* and *Babe*, to their hearts' delight. They would also work on the place and occasionally hunt or fish, completely content with their time together. During those happy times, Pop always called John "Partner." John looked back upon those days, remembering his childhood as especially fortunate because of their relationship and the opportunity that he had to celebrate life with Pop on the Cha Mar.

John and Pop did not capture their time on the Char Mar with a camera. They were too busy living, working and playing in the present. But the happy memories were indelibly printed in their minds' eye and captured by John's poem. Not only does his poem honor his grandfather specifically, but it also points to something else that was John's hallmark. He valued relationships with family members and friends more than anything else.

Partners

*There is more to hunting and fishing
Than bearing a rifle or pole,
It is something you share with another,
It is something that touches your soul.
You hunt and fish with a partner,
You share more than the game.
Your partner you chose to be with
And he chose you the same,
To talk, to whisper, to laugh and cry,
To plan ahead and wish,
To dream and wonder and be concerned,
To try to catch that fish.
To meet in the road after a long day's hunt
In the black curtain of night
With your imagination running wild,
The dark playing tricks with your sight.
And when the sun sinks low in the West
And the lake becomes live with fire,
The time that is shared is more the goal,
Than the meat you put on the fire.
You see, there is honor in hunting and fishing
Honor in the things that are shared.
It is honor that makes two partners
Become a life long pair.*

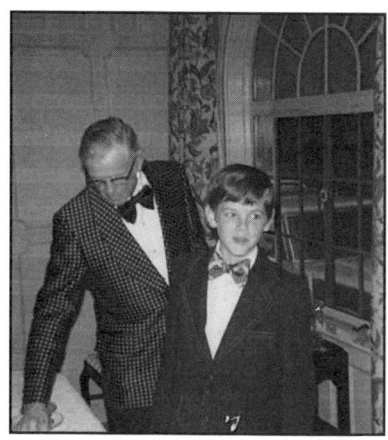

The "Partners" away from the Char Mar and dressed up for the Cotton Palace in Waco where Sally was the duchess from San Antonio, sponsored by her Great Aunt and Uncle, Margaret and Buzz Stevens.

In another poem that I saved, John reflected upon the ominous event that had turned his life from the typical pursuits of young men during their college years to the sober and lonely pursuit of trying to beat the virtually impossible odds of a highly malignant brain tumor.

<u>Reflections on Having a Brain Tumor</u>
*What do you do when life leaves you stranded,
stranded through no fault of your own?
The world spins along and lives are expanded,
but you can't bet on the cards you've been shown.
The moss grows up around your bones and
roots you to the ground.
You wish for lights, colors and song, but never hear a sound.
It's said so much you must not lose hope.
So what do you do when you've run out of rope?
Tie a knot and hang on.*

And that is precisely what John did. By January of '85, the bone infection finally seemed to be under control, so John returned to A&M for the spring semester. Again, he took a full semester of course work, which kept him busy most of the time. When he had the chance, he would take his fishing tackle and go to Lake Somerville for an outing. Another time, only once, he ventured out to the Big Thicket by himself, and almost got hopelessly lost in this wilderness that he had underestimated. But of course, he made it home to tell the story! His first trip home that semester was at Easter. The bone infection had not returned, and John's general health continued to improve as the time lengthened since finishing chemotherapy and having the series of surgeries that continued to interrupt his schooling. We had a joyful Easter with Sancy and Bea returning for the first time since they had stayed with John in the fall. Sally, Jeff (not in picture), West, his wife Dana and their first born son, Matthew, also joined us for the celebration. It is easy to see from the photo, how much better John was feeling and that he was putting on some needed weight!

In the summer of '85, John took time off from school and so we decided to take him on a trip to the Club Med resort in Puerta Vallarta, Mexico. John and I were there for two weeks. Bob, Scott and Rene joined us for the first week. John enjoyed the experience with family, as well as some of the activities such as snorkeling, sailing a small rented boat, and finding a couple of other young men with whom he played basketball on a court at the resort. However, this type of vacation was not as much to his liking as one that would offer more opportunities for "roughing it," that is to hunt, fish or just to commune in nature. As he recovered, he was fortunate to have those opportunities as well, often going on such excursions with his father, brother, or friends to destinations from central to south Texas.

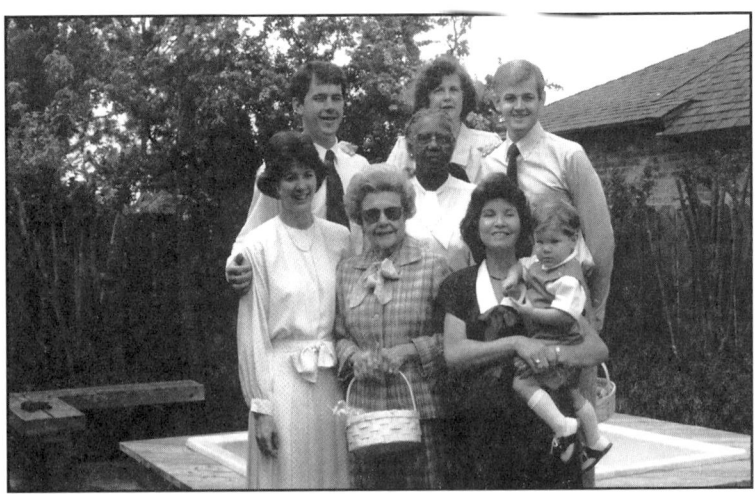

Front row: Sally, Sancy, Dana and baby Matt; second row: West, Bea, John with me in the back

With summer over and John's recovery on track, he once again went back to A&M. This time he and Beaux moved into a small rent house with his brother-in-law's brother, David Jackson. David was there to get a Ph.D. in food science. Finally John' efforts at balancing the treatment for the brain tumor and bone infection with completing his undergraduate work came to fruition. By the time he graduated in May, 1986, John had accumulated many more hours than he needed for a degree, but many of them were for courses taken in the business school at the University of Texas before he transferred to A&M and changed his major to Petroleum Engineering.

What a triumph to graduate in the face of all of the odds that had conspired against him! His family and many friends were there to celebrate the occasion with him. *Beaux* celebrated by stealing and eating much of John's decorated carrot cake. *Beaux* took it from the table to a safe corner of the room, where he ate cake complete with decorations that included an oil derrick artfully drawn with icing. The good news was that he didn't get sick from it, and he left enough for the rest of us to get a small piece!

Now it was time to begin searching for an entry level job as a petroleum engineer. The times could not have been worse for this pursuit because the oil industry was in a severe depression. After looking

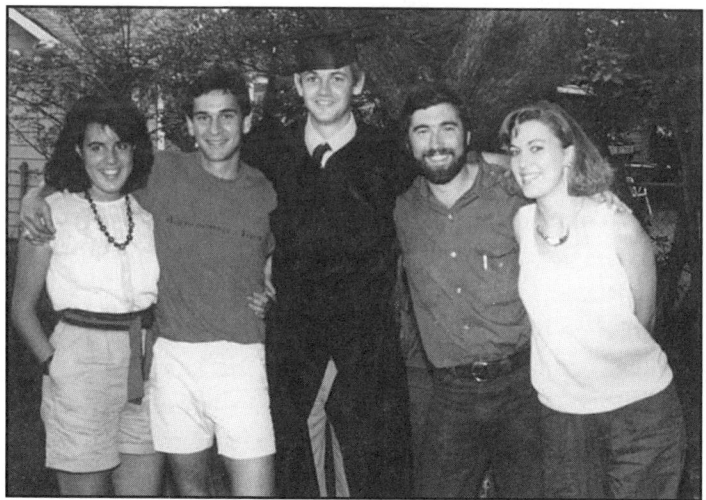

John's friends helping him celebrate graduation from TAMU

for petroleum engineering work all summer in San Antonio, Houston and Dallas, John was persuaded by me to return to A&M. With his foundation in engineering, he decided to take some courses toward a second degree in mechanical engineering, since petroleum engineering at this point seemed futile. I strongly encouraged him to do this, and in retrospect realize that it was a mistake. It was quite reasonable that John was just plain tired of being in school, under the difficult circumstances of his brain tumor, which already had drawn out his years in school from what would have been five years to seven years. At this point he was very unhappy going back to A&M. On top of that, his faithful dog *Beaux*, his constant companion since age 16, died suddenly during the semester of post graduate work. Under these circumstances, John had his worst ever semester academically. He decided not to continue work on a second degree. He wanted to get on with his life! We welcomed him home at the end of the semester in December, and once again, he started his job search. The oil industry was still laying off, not hiring, petroleum engineers. But John was able to find work in environmental engineering. In this field, he could use his knowledge and skills applied to drilling for oil, in order to drill for contaminated water and soil. He would receive "on the job training" in the small company that initially hired him, since the owner of the company had his Ph.D. in geology and was well suited to mentor him. So by early 1987, John was employed as an environmental engineer. He stayed with this firm for about four years before taking a similar job with a larger engineering firm, Weston Solutions, Inc. Soon after taking his first job, he rented an apartment in Sugar Land, and began to date a little as his confidence grew that he would stay cancer free.

  John continued to stay well and free of any signs of recurrence in the fifth summer after his diagnosis and surgery. Therefore, Bob and I took him on a family trip to Santa Fe. Sally had planned the trip. She and husband Jeff, along with Sancy, were with us as well. John had a good time fishing, playing a little golf with Jeff, and enjoying the beautiful country in the Santa Fe area. He joined in the spirit of things by stringing Indian beads to take to his new girl friend. Before he had a chance to give them to her, however, they quit seeing each other, so he ended up giving them to the next girlfriend! We teased him just a little bit about that!

After returning home from Santa Fe, John found a stray puppy on a country road one day, brought her home to the apartment, and named her "Bell." When his first year's lease on the apartment was nearing expiration, he started house hunting. After all, John and his dog needed a yard to enjoy, a garage for his car, his boat and his workshop. As good luck would have it, he found a small old house in the original section of Sugar Land. It was one of numerous small houses built early in the 20th Century for factory workers at the Imperial Sugar plant. When he spotted it (with mother in tow), it caught our collective "eye." It was the right size for a bachelor and it was being thoroughly remodeled. On top of that it was "historical" and much more unique than small tract houses for sale or rent that were spreading like "wild fire" across the prairie. New windows, a new roof, new wiring, refinished floors, remodeled kitchen, paint and new garage door added to its feel of a "brand new" old house! The remodeler and seller was named "Clark Gable." What could be better than that? John ended up buying the house for $45,000, making his down payment from money that he had saved. Then he lived in it for less per month than he had rented his apartment, while enjoying it much, much more.

Now in his new home, he could spend many free hours in his workshop, where he made a canoe and began what became his favorite hobby, primitive bow making. As time passed he became more and more interested in bow making, taking the magazines *Primitive Archer* and *Traditional Bowhunter* in order to learn more and connect with others who had this interest. He continued this hobby for the rest of his life and made many bows, carefully selecting his wood and artfully proceeding with the craft of bow making. He would occasionally have the chance to bow hunt in the Texas hill country with his brother, father or friends. He preferred hunting with his bow than with a gun, and certainly found it to be more of a challenge. He enjoyed all aspects of bow making. Not the least of these was finding the best hard wood to use. He would keep his eyes open all of the time looking close to home, in the country side or where he traveled. As a result, he learned a lot about most of the trees in Texas. His favorite hardwood for bow making was the wood from the Osage-Orange or "bodark" tree. This wood is exceedingly hard and strong. It was prized by the Indians for making bows and war clubs. John prized it too.

Settled in Sugar Land with his new job and home, John's cancer remission continued. He discovered that the several young women that he initially dated after returning to Sugar Land were a way to "bide time" until he met the love of his life, Lisa Beckerdite. It was not long after settling into his new home that he met her. She brought meaning to his life as never before. With her, he found the joy that he had hoped and prayed for against all odds.

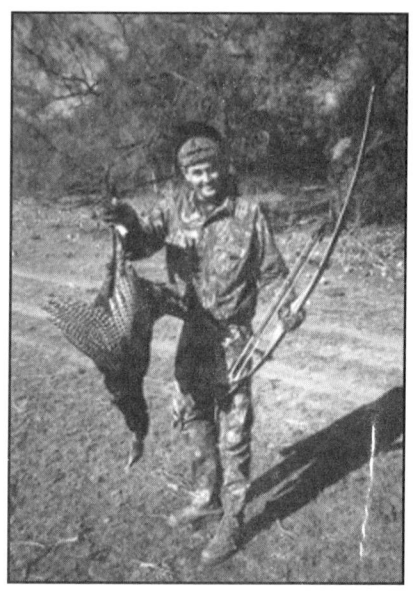

A successful bow hunt with West, who took the snapshot

It all began when Lisa and John met on a night in the fall of 1989. They were both attending an interchurch singles group that was meeting at First United Methodist Church in Sugar Land. Lisa had brought the ice cream for the group. She was trying to retrieve the sizable containers from her car when John drove up in his new white Chevy pick up truck, got out, introduced himself, and offered to carry the ice cream into the church for her. That night was the beginning of a friendship and love that would be the fulfillment of John's life.

Their first date was to the Houston symphony. Bob and I had given John the tickets, and so he asked Lisa to go with him. They ate across from Jones Theatre at Biaporette's Italian Restaurant. Lo and behold! When it was time to pay for the meal, John discovered that he had left his wallet on the dashboard of the car. He woefully realized that he had removed it from his pocket to pay for parking and had failed to put it back into his pocket. Lisa came to the rescue and covered the tab for their dinner! They had many laughs about their first date as their friendship grew into love and then to commitment.

John told Lisa of his medical history and of the serious risk that

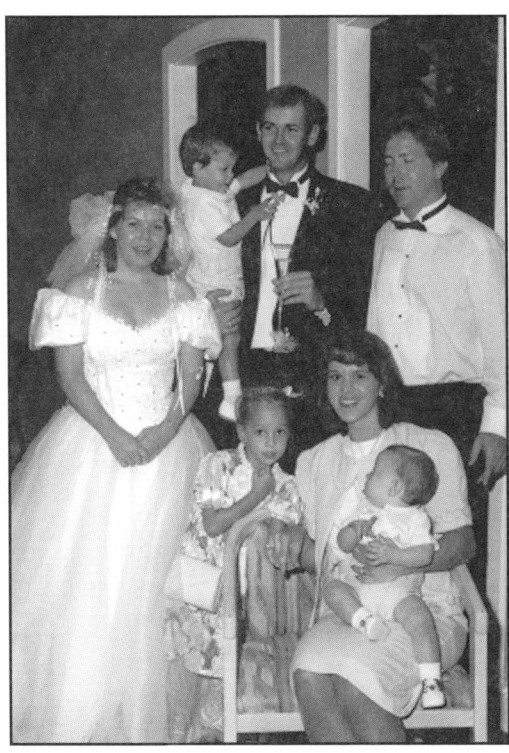

John and Lisa on their wedding day with Ashby and Joanie McMullan and family

his brain tumor would recur. She loved him enough to accept that risk. Thus their plans were made for marriage less than a year after they met. They set the date for their wedding, August 18, 1990. Lisa and her mother planned a beautiful wedding followed by a reception and banquet. Hearts were happy that day as we celebrated the glorious miracle of John's healing, seven years with the cancer in remission and now a wedding. John and Lisa were given a warm send off from family and friends, as they departed for a honeymoon in San Francisco and the wine country.

Not long after returning home from their honeymoon to the "bachelor" house, Bob and I received a phone call. Lisa was pregnant! While she had not expected it so soon, they were thrilled and eager to get their family started. John and Lisa were 29. There was no need to wait. In retrospect, Lisa is confident that God's hand was in their meeting, marriage and family, including the rapidity in which all of these most important events of their lives took place. In the back of John's mind, as the Reverend Dr. Tom Pace later observed, John had learned to "number his days." Perhaps I am the only one who noticed on the day of their wedding, that in the midst of all of the joy that I could see on John's face, his voice broke when the pastor asked him to repeat after him; *I will keep you only unto me ....until death do us part.*

Mary Kaitlin was born on her dad's 30th birthday, June 3,1991. What a wonderful birthday gift. He and Lisa were so thrilled. Mary Kaitlin's arrival brought much joy to their lives. I remembered back when at age 23, about eight months after his brain tumor surgery, John was sent to a new doctor, a radiologist, for a CAT scan. When the doctor was questioning John, he asked his age. When John replied 23, the doctor said rather sadly, "Twenty three, trying to make it to 24." John quickly responded; "No, I'm planning to live to see my grandchildren some day. Now, his dream was just beginning to unfold, as he held his beautiful new baby girl.

John and Lisa had the "bachelor" house converted to meet their immediate needs for bringing home and welcoming their new baby, but they soon realized that they needed more room than their tiny home provided. Again they were lucky in finding a larger house in old Sugar Land. They sold the "bachelor" house for a nice profit, and bought their second home in time for Carly's arrival 2 1/2 years after

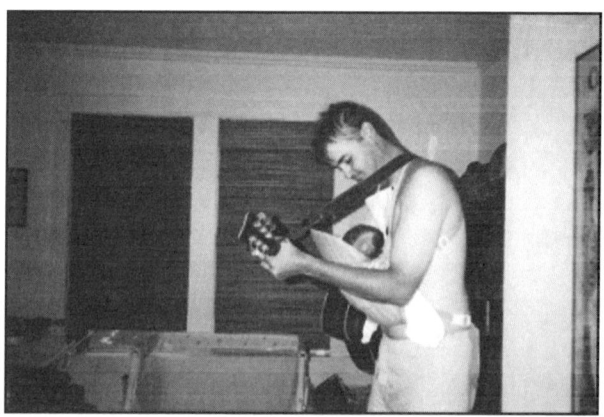

John serenading Mary Kaitlin soon after she arrived home.

Mary Kaitlin. Carla Jane was born on December 21, 1993, which is her grandfather Warren's birthday. Only two months before her birth, her grandfather Carl Beckerdite had died after a long, and for many years, successful battle against colon cancer. Before his death, he was told that his second granddaughter would be named Carla for him and I was told that she would be named Jane for me.

The year after Carly's birth, in 1994, John had an opportunity to move back to San Antonio where his company, Weston Solutions, had opened a new office. He had long dreamed of going home again, so he and Lisa decided to make the move. They lived there for approximately five years. During that time, they bought a small home in the Alamo Heights neighborhood near his childhood home and close to his brother's home and his father's home. There, he enjoyed many happy times with Lisa and the girls at his side, and with many opportunities for all of them to visit his father, stepmother, brother and grandmothers. His old friends quickly drew him and Lisa back into their circle for all kinds of activities, fun and fellowship. They joined a neighborhood church, St Andrews Methodist Church, where Lisa worked in the church office and pre-K school and where they were active members. John coached Mary Kaitlin's first soccer team in San Antonio. Their times there were very happy.

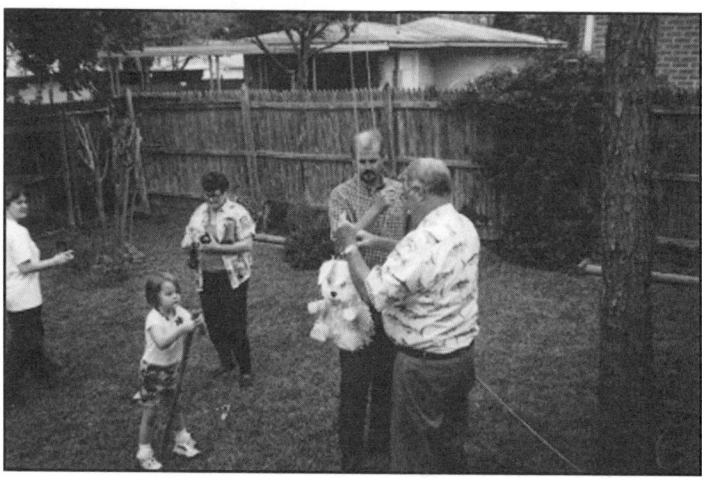

*John and his dad work on an Easter piñata
while Carly and grandmother Charlotte assist*

Nevertheless, during their fifth year in San Antonio, they made the decision to move back to Sugar Land after inquiring with the Houston office and finding that they would like to have him return. They reasoned that Sugar Land was half way between their cities of origin, San Antonio and Shreveport, and that it would be easier to travel from there to both destinations. They had met and lived in Sugar Land, and they knew that they felt at home there. Friends and family were there as well as in their hometowns. And so they returned, much to the delight of their Sugar Land/ Houston family – mother, stepfather and stepsister.

With the selling of their San Antonio home, they purchased a home in Sugar Land's First Colony, relocating in June, 1999. In August, Mary Kaitlin entered the third grade at Colony Bend elementary school and Carly started kindergarten there. John had to finish up about six months of work in San Antonio before he could join them full time in Sugar Land. The family endured unwanted separation during the weekdays, but on weekends they were back together. Near or apart, Lisa and John were devoted to one another and to their girls. John loved to play with his girls. He loved to serenade them with his guitar. He loved to tell them bed time stories, weaving events and pets from his boyhood into his imaginative stories. He, along with Lisa, encouraged their participation in soft ball, soccer, basket ball and swimming, often coaching them actually or in terms of

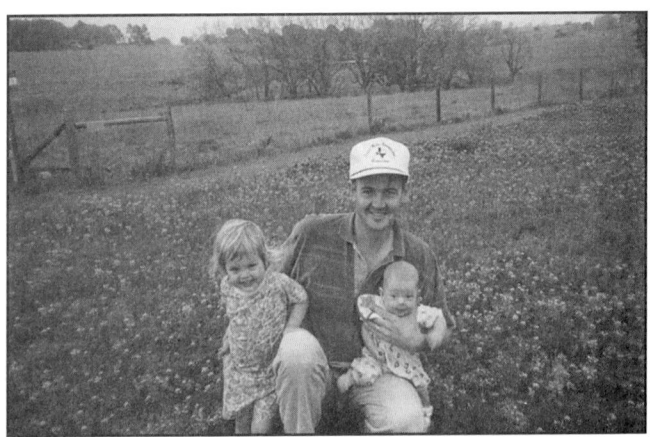

Lisa's photo of John and the girls on a spring day in a field of bluebonnets

advice given. Mary Kaitlin and Carly loved all of those moments with their dad, but he loved them even more.

Back in Sugar Land, they became active in Christ United Methodist Church, which was within walking distance of their new home. They involved their girls in the church as well, serving as acolytes and singing in the children's choir. Always, their family celebrated life and its seasons, playing in fall leaves, and rejoicing in fields of spring bluebonnets. In summer they took vacations traveling to reunion destinations in Texas such as San Antonio, Dallas, Marlin, Lorena and the Bosque River Valley. They attended other reunions held in Louisiana, Arkansas, Maryland, and Oregon. In the winter, they would spend time during their Christmas vacation visiting family in Texas and Louisiana. At all times, they valued and enjoyed their extended family ties. Wherever they lived, they made the most of the days and years together, living life to its fullest. They seemed to learn in a relatively short period of time what really matters in life. Lisa and John insisted that they never had an argument. They certainly never doubted their love or commitment to each other and their girls. They had much joy and happiness.

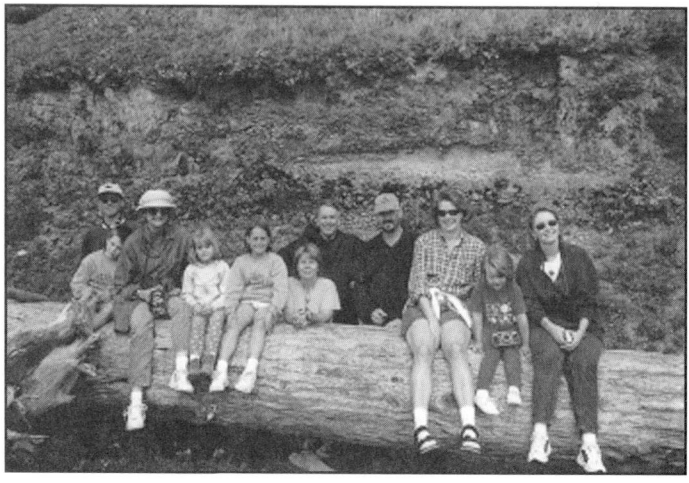

Stevens Family Reunion in Oregon, 1996

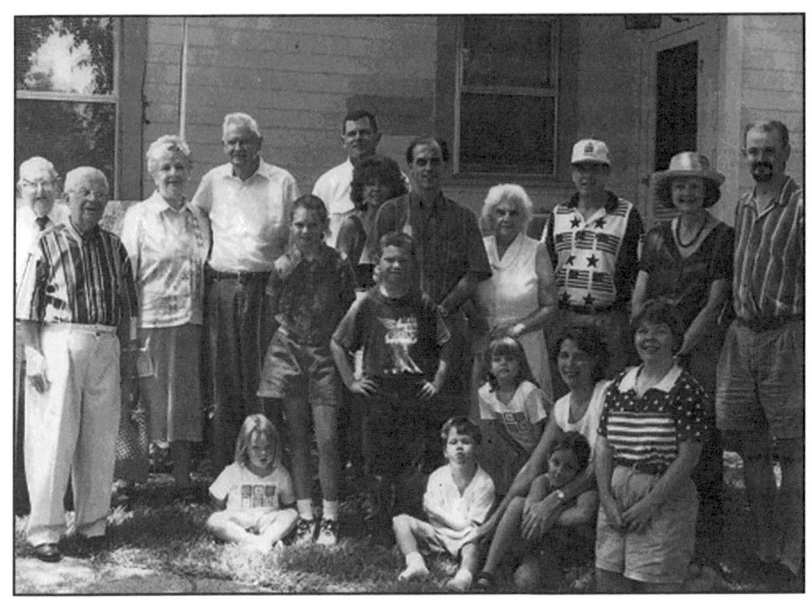

Celebrating July 4, 1997 in Lorena at the Westbrook family reunion.

CHAPTER 3

DIFFICULTIES TO OVERCOME

"Cure me and I will give you my Moses stick!"

John and Lisa were always there for each other in the hard times as well as the happy times. The former seemed to come too soon and too often. Just a short time after they settled into married life and found out that they would be parents the next June, John had a *grand mal* seizure. We were all fearful that the tumor was back and rejoiced when the doctors said that the seizure was attributed to damage from surgery and prior treatment of the tumor that was still in remission. John had also recently taken a blow on his forehead, while hammering in his workshop. The self inflicted blow to his head may have contributed to having the seizure. In any event, for the rest of his life, John would be required to take anti seizure medication.

Between Mary Kaitlin and Carly's birth, Lisa was diagnosed with Stage 1 (relapsing and remitting) multiple sclerosis. Now she and John would both see a neurologist – usually the same one. They joked about it and said that they should get "two (visits) for the price of one," when they would go to the neurologist together. Lisa's father died about three years after their marriage and two years following her MS diagnosis.

One day during the weeks after Lisa and John had made the decision to move from San Antonio back to Sugar Land, but before they had actually made the move, I received a long distance call from Lisa. She was frightened and in tears. She told me that John had been suffering some scary symptoms. They had a visit scheduled with the neurologist seeing him at the time, Dr. Michael D. Merrin. Dr. Merrin had followed his case since 1996, when his previous neurologist in San Antonio had retired. His report filed on the day of John's visit and examination explains more about his symptoms.

March 26, 1999
Re: John Warren

Complicated Migraine (Migraine with Aura)
> *Mr. Warren had an episode that started out with a clear area near the center of his vision and progressed to a left field defect. He did not test each eye individually with this, but I think it probably was bilateral by the way he describes it. He states that he then had some numbness of his left arm and had a little trouble using it without looking at where it was going. Then he developed a headache that was briefly severe and then milder and he had a headache yesterday morning. He had a little bit of the visual symptoms today. He has had this back in grade school, but it has been very intermittent occurring many years apart each time. His neurological examination today does not show any problems and I obtained an MRI scan of the brain which shows the old tumor bed where it was treated both surgically and with radiation therapy, but no evidence of any new tumor or mass effect. An EEG done today was normal. I am going to have him continue on Dilantin, 300 mg. on odd number days and 400 mg on even number days and keep a record of his headaches and contact me in about a month so we can see how he is doing. He may be in a period where he is going to have more headaches.*

<u>Right Temporal Astrocytoma, S/P Total Removal Without Evidence of Recurrence and Secondary Seizure Disorder, Nocturnal.</u>
> *Note above I will see him back again in six months for reassessment.*
> *MDM/gm*
> *Addendum: Mr. Warren may be moving back to Houston and he will either reestablish with Dr. Hauser, or since he is going to live southwest (of Houston) he may go into Dr. Devere or Dr. Martin.*

My heart was in my throat until we received Dr. Merrin's report. Then John and Lisa and all of their loved ones were greatly relieved to hear that there was no indication that the brain tumor had recurred. In the months that followed John's life returned to normal, that of a busy young man with a demanding job, who was relocating with his family to a new home in Sugar Land.

While he and Lisa started seeing a neurologist for routine medication check ups after they were settled in Sugar Land, apparently John did not report further episodes. In retrospect, I think that it is likely that he continued to have some symptoms, but dismissed them as associated with the migraine condition that was diagnosed when he was a boy and again when the symptoms recently reemerged in San Antonio. Thus if further similar episodes occurred, John must not have thought that they were caused by a new brain tumor and thus did not report them to anyone. John was stoic and would tend to think that relatively mild symptoms were something that he could live with. I believe that the timing of the episode in San Antonio was unfortunate in coinciding with the move back to Sugar Land. If it had happened after he returned to Sugar Land, or if he had not moved from San Antonio, perhaps there would have been a six month follow up and more as the San Antonio doctor had recommended. As it happened, when John returned to Sugar Land, no "routine" MRI was scheduled in the next four years. Another factor in John's mind that may have kept him and his new doctors in Sugar Land from being more vigilant, was that John had become unaccustomed to having MRI scans. In this context, Dr. Merrin had written the following report on January 26, 1999, when John visited his office for medication review. Even though John was free of symptoms, he advised John to resume a schedule of routine MRI scans.

January 26, 1999
Re: John Warren
<u>*Right Temporal Astrocytoma, SP Total Removal without Evidence of Recurrence, and Secondary Seizure Disorder, Nocturnal:*</u>
> *Mr. Warren is doing well. It has been a number of years since he has had an MRI scan and we discussed getting one at least every 5 years to make sure the astrocytoma does not come back. He clearly has no symptoms or signs of it now. His one seizure was nocturnal and was in about 1991. He remains on Dilantin, 300 mg on odd numbered days, 400 mg on even numbered days. He has no signs of medication difficulty. He has venous pulsa-*

tions in his fundi and his neurological examination remains normal. If he would like to have an MRI scan anytime in the next year before he comes back to see me, he can call and we can arrange for this. I am encouraging it. A CBC will be obtained and I will see him back in one year.
MDM/gm

Of course as previously indicated, John did return in two months and an MRI scan was done at that time. Hindsight is always 20-20, but if John's story gets across to patients, their families, and their doctors the importance of maintaining vigilance even after 10 or 20 years of remission of glioma brain tumors, then John's story will be of help to others with this lethal form of cancer. One of the neurologist's who was on John's case in 1983, told us *"it was not a matter of if, but a matter of when the cancer would return."* With the glorious passage of so many years without a recurrence, John and all of his family, including me, had become overly optimistic that the neurologist ominous prediction in 1983 no longer applied.

About six years after Lisa's father's death, and soon after John, Lisa and the girls returned to Sugar Land, Lisa lost her mother. John had loved his mother in law and father in law from the beginning, and that never changed. He and Lisa did what they could when Mrs. Beckerdite was stricken with inoperable, metastasized tumors in her brain. They brought her from Shreveport for consultation at M.D. Anderson, but even this great center for the treatment of cancer could not really offer her any treatment or hope. Lisa and John looked after her in their home for much of the short period of time that she lived after her diagnosis. Through all of their difficulties, John worked hard for his company, consulting and doing all that he could as a consultant to solve the problems associated with environmental clean ups on many job sites over the state of Texas and sometimes out-of-state. His company could always depend on him in the good times and the bad ones.

During the stressful times of moving, followed by Lisa's mother dying, John and Lisa both set aside their own health care issues. John no doubt forgot about the advice given by Dr. Merrin to start having routine MRI's. Lisa's stress and grief over her mother's illness and death must have contributed to the beginning of a steady progression of her MS from Stage 1 to Stage 2 (Progressive) as diagnosed in the fall of 2002.

Then on Friday, Jan. 31, 2003, John came home from work early after experiencing what we later learned was a focal seizure in his left arm. He and Lisa went to the Memorial Southwest Hospital Emergency Center. Lisa did not call us until after the ER doctor had sent John for a CAT scan because John did not want her to call us. In his customarily selfless way of living, he didn't want "to put Mother through this again." But Lisa finally insisted and called Bob and me. We immediately went down to stay with them. The ER doctor returned to John's room several hours after the CAT, with the report from the radiologist. The report focused for the most part on the old tumor site from John's first brain tumor, and found no sure evidence of a new tumor. The report indicated that what he saw could be scar tissue, perhaps hemorrhagic material, or possibly a tumor. He recommended that we see a neurologist on Monday. For the next year and eight months, we would all be "put through" great agony, but none so much as John and none with so much courage as John.

On Monday, Feb.3, John and Lisa saw Dr. Herbert Edmondson. Dr. Edmondson had not seen him before. John and Lisa had been planning to make appointments with him, since the previous neurologist that they were seeing in Sugar Land was no longer available to them because of a change in health insurance. Dr. Edmondson reviewed the CAT scan that had been done at the emergency room and then gave John the customary office neurological examination. Overall John's neurological evaluation indicated that he was healthy and normal. Here are excerpts from his medical report pertaining to that day's examination.

> *Patient is awake, alert, and oriented times 3, no evidence of language dysfunction. Fluency, comprehension, naming and repetition are intact, insight is good, demonstrates fluent thinking, judgment is appropriate, there is no disturbance of mood and affect, knowledgeable of current events and past history. Vocabulary is normal, normal attention and concentration.*

Dr. Edmondson saw no evidence of tumor at the old craniotomy location based upon the CAT scan that had been done during his emergency room visit over the weekend. Nevertheless, because of his previous medical history and recent incident of numbness and uncontrollable twitching activity of the left hand and upper extremity, Dr. Edmundson ordered an MRI before we left his office, and he indicated that he would see John after the MRI and other studies were completed.

On Tuesday, Feb. 4, John had his MRI. He did not hear from the doctor's office for the rest of the week. That weekend, Bob and I went to College Station to visit Bob's brother and sister-in-law, Ben and Shirley White, arriving on Friday, and returning home on Saturday. While there, I talked to Shirley about what had happened to John, and I told her that we were waiting on a report from the MRI. I expressed a fair amount of confidence that the MRI would be negative, since the CAT scan had revealed no tumor and since we had not already heard from the doctor.

But on Monday, Feb.10, I was driving to a women's bible study at our church, when my cell phone rang. It was Lisa. She was in tears as Dr. Edmondson's office had called to tell her that she and John must come in today. She was trying to reach John as he was in the field consulting on a project. Though he did not have his cell phone on, she was able to reach him through his office. Lisa and John knew what news the doctor would have for them, otherwise a telephone call would have been sufficient.

After Lisa called me, I called Bob, and then we went in separate cars from different locations to Dr. Edmondson's office in the Neurology Center. Dr. Edmondson told Lisa and John the terrible news first. It was a malignant brain tumor. Then outside the examining room where we were waiting, Bob and I were told. At that time, Dr. Edmondson said to Bob and to me that the tumor was "nasty." I asked him if it was operable. He said he was only sure that it was "biopsable." After that, he took us to John and Lisa in the examining room to discuss treatment alternatives together as a family. The pending biopsy and the possibility of surgery were discussed immediately. Arrangements were made for us to see Dr. John Berry, a well known and reputable neurosurgeon, who had offices at the same

Neurology Center. We went from Dr. Edmondson's office straight to Dr. Berry's office. Arrangements were put in motion for a biopsy to be scheduled as soon as possible.

Compounding our horror at what was unfolding, the next day on Tuesday, Feb.11, Bob heard from his doctor, Dr.Bryan Miles, that he had early prostate cancer. When we went to the doctor's office, he advised surgery. Now this had to be coordinated with John's surgery. Ultimately, Bob's surgery was set for two weeks after John's scheduled surgery.

John had a biopsy at the Southwest Memorial Hospital on Tuesday, Feb. 18. Even this procedure which invaded his brain was scary for us, to say nothing of our fear over what would be found. At best the doctor thought, and we were hoping, that the tumor would be a slow growing tumor, grade 1 or 2, rather than grade 3. Our hopes were dashed when the final biopsy results from the frozen section received the next week indicated Anaplastic Astrocytoma Grade III. This was the same type and grade that John had had 20 years before, but in a different location. Our only "good news" was relative. The new tumor, described as about the size of a golf ball, was "only" 1/2 the size of the first tumor.

We were all shocked that the brain tumor had happened at all after John had been tumor free for nearly 20 years. The doctor's best guess was that it was not the same tumor of 20 years before, since so much time had passed and it was in a different location. The 1983 tumor had been in the right frontal lobe. The new tumor was in the right parietal lobe near the motor strip. The old tumor was 6cms x 4cms, roughly the size of a peach, and the new tumor was determined to be 3cms x 2cms, roughly as previously noted, the size of a golf ball. However, the definitive biopsy from the frozen section which proved the tumor to be the same kind and grade as before, did not prove one way or another whether this was a new tumor or a recurring tumor. In any event, the treatment the doctors chose would be the same. Nevertheless, we felt, and the doctors seem to imply, that if the tumor was new rather than a recurrence, John's chances of survival improved slightly. We did not know it then, but unlike the history of the first tumor, we rarely had any good news to come over the next year and eight months.

Since the Astrocytoma Grade III was a faster growing tumor

than at first had been expected, plans were speeded up for surgery. It was scheduled for March 5. From our perspective, even this was too long to have to wait. The surgery would now take place 3 1/2 weeks from first learning that a tumor had been found and 4 1/2 weeks from his presenting symptom.

On March 5, John had his surgery at St. Luke's hospital. Dr. Berry chose to operate at St. Luke's because of the new guidance system that they had in place that improved the accuracy of brain surgery. This was the second brain tumor surgery in John's lifetime. His first tumor had been excised nearly 20 years before on July 14, 1983. This time, he came through the surgery much better, all things considered. The tumor was not as large or as deep into his brain as the first tumor. Also, the technology for brain surgery was greatly improved and included imaging with a new guidance system that was unheard of 20 years before.

In addition to getting the entire "gross" tumor, Dr. Berry put Gliodel Wafers into the tumor site before closing John's incision. This was a relatively new treatment, officially approved at this point only for Glioblastoma, Grade IV. He had coordinated this treatment with Dr. Morris Groves at M.D. Anderson, who would be John's oncologist after the surgery.

While John was in intensive care, Dr. Berry showed the post surgery MRI's to Lisa and me. He pointed out the proximity of the tumor site to the motor strip on the right side of his brain. He said that he would have liked to extend out further to remove additional tissue that probably had microscopic cancer cells, but he did not want to take a chance on damaging the motor strip, which could leave John impaired with partial paralysis. He hoped that chemotherapy would kill the remaining cells, but he added; "If we have to, we can go back in."

During this surgery and hospitalization, as with the surgeries to follow, our minister Tom Pace and other members of our community of faith came to see John prior to and after surgery to give him support and to pray. All of our family gathered to pray and wait, except his beloved daughters who stayed at home with their step grandmother Charlotte taking care of them until John recovered enough for them to come to the hospital to see him and beg him to hurry home.

After the first surgery, as in all brain surgery, John was in the Intensive Care Unit for several days. However because they had no private room available, they kept him in ICU longer than needed. After being in the hospital for only three days, John was sent home directly from the ICU unit. He had exceeded Dr. Berry's expectations in terms of his recovery time. Back home, Lisa and John were supported by friends, neighbors and church groups bringing food and extending prayers and well wishes – a pattern that would continue through all of his hospitalizations and crises with the disease. " All in all, John and the rest of us felt very hopeful and even optimistic at this point in time. In the spirit of that optimism, I went to our local Asian market and bought some miso paste and other ingredients that we would need in order for John to adhere to a macrobiotic diet, as he had done in 1983.

On March 10, John visited Dr. Groves at MD Anderson for the first time. Lisa, Bob and I went with him. Lisa and John already knew Dr. Groves and liked him. He was the MDA doctor that had been consulted during Lisa's mother's short illness with the metastasized tumor to the brain. John posted in his journal the following summary of what we learned on the first visit to Dr. Groves' office.

> *Dr. Groves discussed post surgery options, especially chemotherapy versus radiation. His concerns were based upon damage from previous radiation and chemotherapy that was done to the veins and arteries. He indicated that my case was so unusual and complicated that the MDA Tumor Board was reviewing it to determine whether or not radiation would be feasible.*

Then Bob had his prostectomy at the Methodist Hospital on March 12. We were expecting an uneventful surgery that would last about 3 hours. Instead, his surgery lasted about 8 hours. Dr. Miles had touched an unusually large and vulnerable vein in his attempt to remove the prostate gland using a prostescopic procedure. Bob lost 9 pints of blood in the process, which were replaced by transfusions. Because of this unexpected problem, Dr. Miles had to abandon this newer, less invasive procedure and open Bob the "old fashion" way. It was a difficult and anxious afternoon, not only for Dr. Miles, but for me as well. The nurse came in time and time again to tell me of the status of the surgery. However, it was not until Bob was finally out of surgery and in intensive care that I realized what a dangerous situation had developed. For most of the night, Bob had a breathing tube to prevent fluid on his lungs. I reluctantly left the waiting area at about 10:00 that evening, as visiting hours were over for ICU. I stayed with my step daughter Rene, whose condominium was only several blocks away from the hospital. When I returned early in the morning, the breathing tube was out and Bob was looking much better. What relief I felt over the positive turn of events. Thankfully, Bob's cancer was removed early, his recovery went smoothly, and all of his subsequent PSA tests have confirmed that he is cancer free.

For John, appointments with Dr. Groves became standard procedure but never routine. For Lisa, Bob and I, it became our standard procedure to be there with him. We worked together as a team, to ask questions, and to use our collective memory, which was better than any individual memory, both in terms of pertinent questions and remembering the answers that we would receive. On our visits, John bantered with Dr. Groves and Dr. Groves, with him. Dr. Groves told John that he had never had a patient who did not complain until John came along. Appointments with Dr. Groves were routinely scheduled a day after the bimonthly MRI. John's father came from San Antonio to join us for some of these appointments, while John's stepmother, Charlotte, would stay at John and Lisa's home to be there for the Mary Kaitlin and Carly when they returned from school or other activities of the moment.

On John's first visit and for many subsequent visits, he brought a walking stick to the MDA clinic that he had hand crafted. It was about four feet tall. He used it because as he walked from place to place, he had difficulty avoiding objects appearing on the left side of his body. This was because of the proximity of the new surgery site to John's motor strip. The condition improved for a while during the months after surgery. But John used his stick for as much and as long as he felt more secure with it.

John loved whittling walking sticks as he loved making bows with the variety of Texas trees and their wood from which he could pick. He had selected this stick carefully. It was made from live oak,

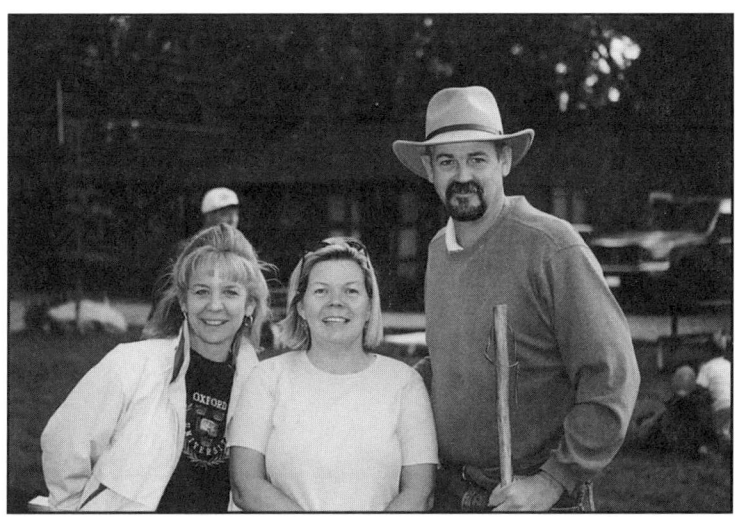

John, Lisa, a friend and the "Moses Stick" on summer vacation after the first surgery in 2003

a beautiful but relatively common tree across Texas. The wood is heavy, hard and strong. John chose a limb that was about 1 1/2 inches in diameter and nearly white with the bark removed. He whittled it until it was smooth. He finished it with a dull luster and topped it off with a leather loop inserted through a hole that he had whittled near the top. He had originally crafted this walking stick for Lisa. But after he began using it, it was soon dubbed the 'Moses stick" by Dr. Groves, and then we all began referring to it in that way. John quipped with Dr. Groves saying; "Cure me and I will give you my Moses stick!" Interestingly enough, strangers in the MD Anderson long hallways, traveling to and from their respective treatments and doctors, also commented on it affectionately, one even calling it a "Moses" stick without knowing that was what we already called it.

On March 13, John's staples were removed by the neurosurgeon. The next day, John was to call Dr. Groves regarding the results of the Tumor Boards' deliberation. He told John that the Tumor Board agreed with Dr. Groves to proceed with limited (pin pointed) radiation therapy before chemotherapy. By the time he told John, Dr. Groves had already put the plan into motion. So on March 14, John had another MRI and more lab work. This was followed by a consultation with the radiologist. However, enough time had to pass from surgery and from insertion of the Gliodel Wafers before the radiation treatment could begin.

With the radiation treatment approaching, I asked Dr. Groves and the MDA nutritionist about the possibility of John going on the macrobiotic diet. The nutritionist advised against it, as there was concern that the high level of antioxidants in the diet would compromise the effectiveness of the radiation and chemotherapy in attacking the malignant cells. So I abandoned the idea of keeping John's home adequately supplied with miso soup and other macrobiotic diet specialties as I had done in 1983.

Radiation began on March 24 and continued through April 25. During this time, John received radiation therapy five days a week. Lisa and I both went with him, sometimes together and at other times alternating our trips with him. Jeff McDonald, associate pastor at our church, regularly scheduled trips to the Medical Center to visit church members. Frequently, he would include a visit to check on John and to visit with Lisa and me as we waited during John's radiation therapy. After the radiation protocol was finished, there was another prescribed waiting period before chemotherapy could begin, which was about six weeks.

During this stressful time, John kept his spirits and his faith strong. In spite of the limitations on treatment for John, given the radiation and chemo that he had had 20 years before, he and the rest of his loved ones continued holding onto their deep seated beliefs that because he had beaten the odds then, he could beat them now. Adding to the strength of that belief was the fact that the new tumor was only one half the size of the first one. We also assumed science must had made significant strides in the treatment and had thus improved success rates in fighting this deadly cancer, even though Dr. Groves had been frank with us about the dismal statistical odds of surviving for five years. And we all knew how much will John had to live and how much faith he had in the healing powers that God instills in us. And so John, with optimism and with his sweet way of finding something to be thankful for in all circumstances, told us that he was thankful that in all of this so far, he did not have pain and most of all, he knew that he was loved.

Over the past year, John, Lisa and the girls had been planning a summer trip to Estes Park, Colorado. It was to begin right after school was dismissed at the end of May. The trip as scheduled would throw the beginning of chemotherapy a couple of weeks later than was absolutely necessary, but Dr. Groves did not think that this would adversely affect the treatment. Thus the two-week trip was taken and all had a good time, though they reported that during the second week they were all getting a little tired and ready to return home. After returning home, there was a "bureaucratic" delay in delivery of the chemotherapy, so his first dose was not started until the first part of July, about nine weeks, instead of six weeks, from his last radiation treatment.

The chemotherapy consisted of Temozolomide for the treatment of recurrent and progressive malignant glioma, combined with Pegylated interferon (Alpha 28/Peg-Intron). Added to the "cocktail" was Tamoxifen, a widely used chemotherapy for breast cancer. This treatment was at that time, the recommended first line of treatment by the National Cancer Institute. It was considered very promising based upon previous clinical trials and research. It had the added benefit, if it worked, of having less severe side effects than most chemotherapy treatments for brain tumors. Each treatment consisted of a 4 week cycle. His first round went relatively well in terms of minimal side effects. John went back to work, drove himself and was able to lead a fairly normal life, even returning to the "field" in October, where much of his engineering consulting work had been done in the past. He continued his first chemo protocol with MRI evaluation occurring every 2 months. His MRI at the end of August was not remarkable. John and all of us remained optimistic.

In many ways, the new cancer brought back memories from the past. He coincidentally found out that Lu Lu, the nurse who had been so kind to him when he was in the Del Oro Hospital twenty years before, was now retired. He also discovered at the same time that she and her husband lived near John and Lisa and that she was in poor health, so he contacted her and went to see her. She had a little trouble remembering him, but with his help she did. I am sure that he tried to encourage her as she had encouraged him so many years ago.

Then two months later after the bimonthly MRI (November 6,

2003), we were shocked again. Dr. Groves reported "little nubbins" or enhancements at the surgical site that were deemed to be cancerous. The Temozolmide chemo regimen was discontinued (after four 4-week courses). With Dr. Groves approval, we immediately made an appointment for November 11 to see the neurosurgeon, Dr. Berry. Lisa and I were heartened in remembering Dr. Berry's comment that we could "go in" again, if necessary. When Dr. Berry saw John's situation, he took action very quickly. The second surgery was scheduled for November 19. After the surgery, when Dr. Berry came to the waiting room, his report left us very apprehensive. He said that while he had gotten the visible tumor, it was a bad one and he knew he was leaving cancer cells that needed to come out, but the cost to John would have been paralysis. Then he said; "The next chemo has to work."

This time, John's recovery from surgery also went smoothly. He was moved to a private room after three nights in ICU. He spent only one more night in the hospital before being released. In that time, we learned the sad news that Dr. Berry's brother, also a physician, had been killed in a motorcycle accident shortly after John's surgery. Afterward, we found out that, possibly due to that tragedy, a routine second MRI was inadvertently omitted before John was released from the hospital. This MRI would have been used later to compare and evaluate progress at the tumor site after bruising and other effects of the surgery itself had receded.

After the second surgery, John could not be given any more radiation. The good news was that since there would be no radiation, there was less delay in starting chemotherapy. Just three weeks after surgery, John was able to start his new chemotherapy, a combination of Cisplatin and CPT-11. It was another clinical trial. There had been concern as to whether or not John would be accepted into this research because he had taken the same thing in another form 20 years ago. Also as previously mentioned, the protocol required that an MRI should have been done after surgery and before release from the hospital. Ultimately, John was approved for the clinical trial as a "special exception." This was done in time to start the treatment the first week in December.

The treatment consisted of infusion therapy given to him as an outpatient at MDA, which was scheduled to be administered for 9 cycles of 4 weeks each. On his first visit of each month, he would spend about 14 to 16 hours at MDA, with both Cisplatin and CPT 11 given to him after hydration. This was the longest procedure. Depending upon the time of day that he was scheduled to begin treatment, John would get home anywhere from 10 PM to 5 AM the next morning. Two subsequent weekly treatments were administered at MDA each month. They consisted of hydration and the CPT-11 infusion only and would take about three hours, if there were no major delays. The fourth week John had no treatment. Nevertheless, it was an exhausting schedule. The treatment drained him as he experienced nausea, some vomiting, loss of appetite and profound tiredness. Yet he remained positive and hopeful. He said that he was glad the treatment caused tangible side effects (including hair loss) because to him that was an indication that it was toxic enough to kill the cancer cells.

Lisa took him for his first treatment of both Cistplatin and CPT-11 in December, and for the subsequent two shorter treatments (CPT 11 only). For the first treatment, they arrived in the afternoon and did not return home until about 2:00 AM the next day. It was clear that for her to continue to take John would be detrimental to her health, given her need for adequate rest to control the progression of MS as well as her need to take care of Carly and Mary Kaitlin. I very willingly offered to take John to MDA for the duration of his treatments, which I began doing with his first treatment in January. I was so thankful for this opportunity to be with him and to support him in this way.

In the meantime Christmas came. On Christmas Eve, we attended a church service and then on Christmas morning, we had a "tree" at John and Lisa's house. Under the tree there was the usual exchange of family gifts. But for Mary Kaitlin and Carly, there were many more gifts given by John's friends and co-workers at his workplace, Weston Solutions. They also gave John and Lisa a generous Christmas gift of money collected from their own pockets as an expression of their love and concern.

The last week in December was the fourth week "break" following John's first round of chemotherapy. Therefore on New Years' weekend, he felt well enough to go with Lisa, the girls, Bob and me to Marlin for the Brazelton/Battle family reunion. This reunion has

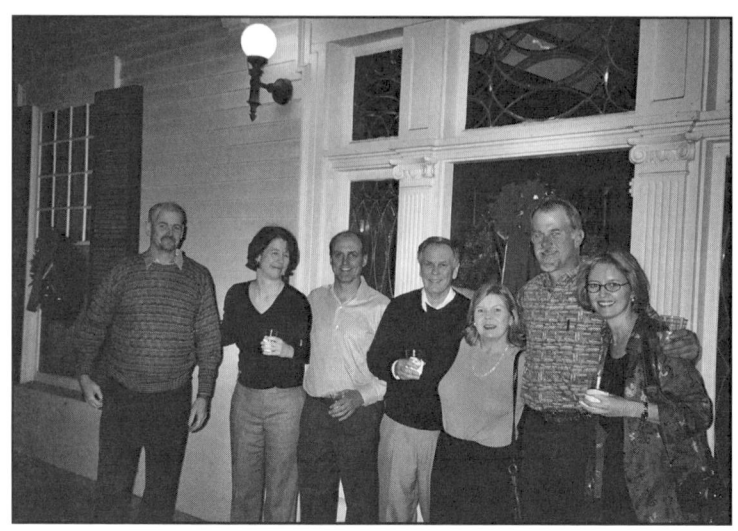

*John, Sally, Jeff, Bob, Lisa, West and Rene
in front of the historic Allen House, Marlin, Texas*

always been special, because our cousins Berry and Chrissie Brazelton have made a tradition of hosting it almost every year during the first week in January. They come from Cambridge, Massachusetts to land that they own in Marlin that was once a part of the Jones/Battle plantation. They invite the rest of the clan to come

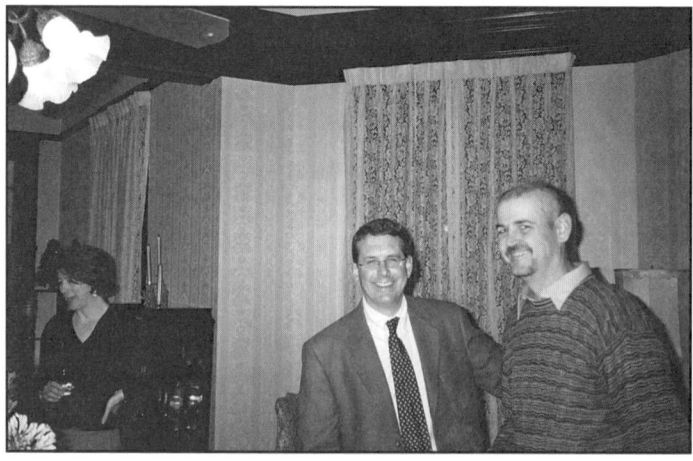

John and his cousin Tom Brazelton enjoying the reunion

from all parts of Texas to enjoy the bond of kinship and shared family history at the Allen House, a historic home that is available to rent for parties. John, Lisa, and the girls had attended many of these reunions in the past. They were especially happy to be able to go this time. West and his youngest son Michael came from San Antonio to the annual event for the first time ever as did Rene. Sally, Jeff, William and Lydia were also there, as they had been for many previous reunions. Here many cousins from our "Battle" side of the family going back to our common ancestor Thomas Elbridge Battle enjoy the holiday food and drink, while visiting and singing along with the piano to back us up. John was feeling well enough to enjoy it a lot.

After the party ended in Marlin, John, West and Michael drove the relatively short drive to his cousin Bill Stevens' ranch near Crawford for a duck hunt the next day. The rest of us drove to Sally and Jeff's country home in the Bosque River Valley near Clifton, and just a few miles from Crawford. The weather was cold and I was very worried about John venturing out for the duck hunt with his immune system weakened by the new chemotherapy. But when they met us later the next day at Sally and Jeff's place, they were all smiles. John had been wrapped up warmly and tucked in a duck blind, where he saw some ducks, and enjoyed himself, though he did not fire a gun.

After the Christmas and New Year holidays, John had his second infusion treatment of Cisplatin and CPT 11 on January 7th, which he noted in his journal. It was increasingly hard to tolerate this highly toxic treatment. The next day he wrote that he had diarrhea, but also recorded that he had completed some work at the office - a four hour effort. I can only imagine how difficult that was for him, but I know how motivated he was to continue to work for the sake of his family. His journal notes also said; "~~I did not want~~ ... he corrected and clarified the statement to read; "I could not eat." His digestive system was very upset by the treatment. Diarrhea continued to be a problem. It became more and more difficult for him to go to his office and to be productive there, yet he persevered. He could no longer go to the field, but would do what office work he could, mostly consisting of writing the health and safety plans for each project as required by law. When the effects of treatment caused him to miss a day, he would worry.

In his January 9 journal notes, he reported that he was "weak and shaky," but on January 13, he reported "feeling better." Then reflecting his struggle and desire to continue, he entered in his journal on January 14 that he had another CPT-11 infusion. This second treatment was not quite as hard on him as the first treatment each month which included Cisplatin. Thus he added; "Maybe (I) could have gone back to work." He was referring to the day after completing the treatment. I believe that this would have been next to impossible as even this relatively "easier" treatment would always weaken him and make him feel worse in a variety of ways.

Each month after the three week course of treatment, he would begin feeling a little better during the fourth week of rest. No sooner than he would feel better, than it would be time to go back for another infusion. However, as the treatment continued, feeling better was relative. His overall condition was getting weaker and less tolerant of the toxic chemotherapy.

In addition, in March, John developed a blood clot. His right leg had been hurting him badly behind his knee for several days before his second infusion treatment of the month (CPT-11 only). This was a "short" infusion day. When the attending nurse heard his complaint, she called the Brain and Spine Center offices. While John thought he had injured his knee, the nurse was very concerned because she knew what we did not know, which was that brain tumor patients are subject to blood clots. At her insistence, we went up to the doctor's office after the infusion treatment was completed. The nurse felt behind his knee, and after reporting to the doctor, John was sent for a Doppler scan which confirmed the blood clot. He was immediately put on Fragmin, which over time would diminish the clot. We were several hours later getting home that night than expected. John and I both were tired and discouraged but still with hope. Ultimately, the clot improved to the point that it was no longer palpable and painful.

Another complication, directly related to the Cisplatin was further loss of hearing. John already had moderate hearing impairment from 20 years ago, when he took Cisplatin the first time. As the hearing difficulties worsened, we began to discuss the possibility of hearing aids. However, the doctors discouraged getting them before the hearing loss (mostly consonants) had peaked or nearly so. In retrospect, I wish that he would have had them sooner, while he was still going to his office so he could have been able to benefit more from them.

Nevertheless, during this difficult time, John maintained his sense of humor. There are many examples. For instance, he had difficulty tucking his shirt in the back because his left hand and arm were not working properly, so when he would get to work with his shirt only partially tucked in, he would get a male co-worker named Vince to tuck it in the rest of the way. He dubbed him "my office wife." He liked to turn the humor on himself when he could not hear. He would do this by taking bits and pieces of someone's remarks that he could hear, and then coming back with a nonsensical statement, usually pretty funny. I wish that I had written some of his quips down for posterity. One that I recall happened one afternoon in the spring of 2004. Lisa drove her car about two blocks to the Middle School to pick up Mary Kaitlin. As luck would have it, a patrol officer stopped her because one of her brake lights was out. Upon further investigation and to make matters worse, the officer found that Lisa did not have her proof of insurance in the car (although she was insured). He also found her inspection sticker was expired. When she returned home with three citations and told John about it, he quipped; "Well Lisa, you should have played the brain tumor card!" Maybe fewer citations would have been issued! Not all comments were humorous. Some were heartrending. As I would drive John to MDA every week for infusion treatments or related appointments on the Southwest Freeway, we would pass an area where day laborers waited in hopes of being hired. John would see them and feel great compassion for them and their plight. Yet he said; "You know Mother, I envy them, for they have their health." My heart was crushed.

John continued the bimonthly MRI's followed by an appointment the next day with Dr. Groves to hear the verdict. If John could tolerate it and the cancer continued to remain in remission, then the protocol was to continue for nine months. John's cancer nurse told us that so far, none of Dr. Groves patients had been able to complete nine months. However, she added to encourage us, one patient had not been taken off until the 8th month. John and I continued to go three weeks with a one week break in between cycles through May.

In March, the tumor site still looked good as there were no visible "enhancements." However, there was a worrisome round spot about the size of a pea in a new area on the left frontal lobe of his brain. The doctor could positively identify the area as hemorrhagic. However, he could not tell what was causing that condition. He could only speculate that since it was near the original 20 year old tumor site, it may have been caused by the impact of the chemotherapy weakening his blood vessels in this area that were already weakened from the massive dose of radiation that he received 20 years before. We knew that the possibility of a new cancer lurking behind the bleeding area could not be completely overruled. This left John and all of us worried. Still, we were relieved that both the original and the new tumor sites did not show new enhancements. Two months later, at the end of May this would all change.

In the meantime, we continued his "routine" schedule of infusion therapy. Sally, West and Rene wanted to be a part of this. So West came in April and Sally, in May, to be with John during the long and most difficult first treatment of each of the cycles, when both Cisplatin and CPT 11 were infused over approximately a 14 hour period. Rene opted to come often to visit during these treatments. They also wanted "Mother" to have a rest from the long hours of the first infusion treatment. Nevertheless, it was difficult for me not to be there for John during those two long, hard treatments when Sally and West were with him. So I went down anyway to stay with John for a few hours during that time.

The Cisplatin treatment continued to produce the worst side effects of all of the treatments that he had endured. He would get a metallic taste in his mouth. Sometimes nausea would cause vomiting, which happened during two of the treatments when I was with him and then again on West's watch. However, he had a less difficult time when Sally was there for infusion therapy, for at least, he did not vomit. I continued to go with him as before, for the infusions of CPT-11 only. During all of the treatments when I went with John, he was stoic, patient and complained very little, although I know that he always suffered from the toxicity of the treatments. He lost weight, something he watched closely, hoping that he would not lose so much weight as he did 20 years before when undergoing chemotherapy. But his appetite was very limited. There were many hospital food selections that he definitely did not like or want while he was taking the infusion treatments, one being a particularly rich and "nasty" gumbo. I found that egg salad sandwiches and turkey sandwiches were pretty well received by him. Generally during infusion therapy and for several days afterward, he would lose his appetite for most foods.

During the months of undergoing the infusions as John and I would sit together, I would long for words that would be comforting to him. Sometimes we prayed together. More often, I prayed silently and I am sure that John prayed silently as well. A few times, I took the Bible and read from it. At other times we would just watch a little TV together, we would read books or magazines, or both of us would sleep as best we could. I began to take my Pilates mat on the long infusion days. I would roll it out on the narrow strip of flooring between his bed and the wall of his cubicle. I would lie there worried and sad but otherwise content just to be by his side. He expressed concern about my lying on a mat on the floor, and wanted me to find a more comfortable solution, but as the night wore on into the early morning hours, it looked and felt pretty good to me.

In May, in order to continue the infusion treatment, a "long line" had to be put in John's left arm because the nurses could no longer find a vein anywhere that was good enough to insert the needle for the infusions. John hated to be stuck over and over again as the nurses would look for a vein to use. This had been going on the entire time that he had been receiving the infusions. As a result, from early in the process, John insisted that specialty nurses be sent in to find the vein and set him up for the infusions. They could avoid most of the repeated stabs that had caused John to leave the hospital with new bruises and puncture wounds every time. So when even the specially trained and experienced nurses could not find a vein, he took the new setback in his stride and accepted the "long line" stoically. However, when the surgeon came to the infusion cubicle and performed the surgery to insert the line, I stood outside the door, looking in as John patiently endured. I wept, but John did not know this. Somehow this turn in events seemed very foreboding to me. I wondered at my son's great courage and patience in the face of such ongoing hardship, suffering and the knowledge of the tremendous odds against him.

My feelings of doom were well founded. John had his routinely scheduled MRI on May 29. The results were ominous. When we met with Dr. Groves on May 30, following the MRI, he told us that there were some significant new enhancements at the tumor site. As always, he had the MRI pictures on a computer screen to show us what he was talking about. However, Dr. Groves also told us that he was about 85% sure that it was necrosis and not a recurrence of the cancer. Part of his reasoning stemmed from the fact that John still performed fairly well on the routine neurological exams given in the office that day. There had not been much change if any from two months ago. However, Dr. Groves wanted John to take a "rest" from the chemo and come back in three to four weeks for another MRI.

In the meantime, John, Lisa, the girls, Bob and I had planned to take a trip to the YMCA Camp at Estes Park from June 12 to June 19. We planned to fly. Jeff and Sally gave enough of their Advantage miles to John, Lisa and the girls to cover their round-trip flight. This really made the trip possible as John was too sick for the pretty but arduous drive. The trip would have coincided with his week "off" if he had been able to receive the 7th course of treatment. With this turn of events, we did not want to delay the next MRI as we felt great anxiety, even in the face of Dr. Groves' cautious optimism. When asked, Dr. Groves indicated that he would make the trip if he were in John's place. So after discussing our trip plans with Dr Groves and questioning the feasibility of it, John and all of us agreed – we would quickly reschedule the trip to leave on June 5 and return on June 12. That way there would be no delay in the follow-up MRI.

Chapter 4

THE LAST SUMMER

"In the fear of the Lord ... one's children will have a refuge."
Proverbs 14.26

Lisa, John and the girls had two previous summers at the Estes Park YMCA camp prior to the summer of 2004. They already knew how much they loved the place. The first summer that they went to the Estes Park YMCA Camp was in 2002. This was before John's diagnosis, and they were still living as most of the young families around them, with joy and confidence that they had many years more to come. When they returned in 2003 after John's initial diagnosis, surgery and radiation therapy, they were still able to make the trip by car. At that time, John and all of us were holding onto hope that once again, as twenty years before, his cancer would go into long-term remission. Also since the radiation that he had between March 24 and April 25 was a minimal and "pin pointed" dose, the side effects had been mild and by the first of June, he was fairly well recovered. He did not start chemotherapy until the first of July, several weeks after they returned home. So the 2003 trip, for the most part, was uneventful from the standpoint of John's tumor. Though the shadow of John's disease was over them, they were able to get by mostly as the year before.

On June 3, 2004, two days before the six of us were scheduled to depart for Colorado, Rene and her friend Houshyar took us for a joint birthday celebration at Cafe Adobe, a festive and popular spot on the banks of Oyster Creek, to celebrate John and Mary Kaitlin's shared birthday. After placing our orders, we were enjoying the atmosphere and each other when John had a seizure. It was a focal seizure that involved not only his left arm and hand as previous seizures, but much of his left side, including his face. He struggled with it for what seemed a long time; we guessed a minute or more, as we all sat helpless to do anything. Lisa was next to him, and calmly comforted him with her gentle pats. I tried to stay calm. Surprisingly, I had never before witnessed John having a seizure, except perhaps for the trembling that I saw while he was in ICU after his 1983 surgery. I agonized for him as I helplessly watched. Before it was over, I got up and walked around the table to touch him in what I hoped was a comforting gesture. Shortly thereafter the seizure had run its course. Once it was over, John looked at us and said quietly and somewhat apologetically, "I couldn't help it." Of course, we all knew that, but this statement coming from him at that time was poignant. It revealed to me how much he longed for some control over the disease. This seizure was a rude awakening as to how formidable the odds had become. I almost cried as my primitive feelings of protectiveness toward my child and my helplessness collided.

John and all of us knew that he should not drive himself to work for his last day before leaving on the trip. So the next morning, June 4th, I picked him up and drove him to his office. I could tell that he was suffering the aftermath of the seizure and was a little confused. The very fact of the seizure began eroding whatever hopes that I had that the enhancement seen in the most recent MRI did not represent a recurrence. I am sure that his unspoken thoughts were the same. Yet we could not know or possibly believe that June 3, his birthday, was the last day that he would ever drive his car.

On June 5, John, Lisa, Mary Kaitlin, Carly, Bob and I left on our Colorado vacation. John continued to be a little confused as our baggage was being checked. In an effort to help, he picked up a bag that had not been tagged and put it on the conveyor belt. It was gone in an instant. I told the sky cap who was checking us in of the mishap. He was very nice, but anxious to get up to the bag's destination, so that he could check it in. In the days since *9/11*, having an unidentified piece of luggage in the system was a major problem. The next confusion occurred when we arrived at our departure gate. It had been changed to another gate in another terminal. In proceeding to our new gate and to our dismay, John walked away from the rest of us and we could not find him. We had his ticket and Lisa had his wallet. I became extremely anxious, thinking that he was possibly disoriented, with no identification in the crowded airport. Lisa, the girls and Bob were anxious too, though perhaps a little calmer than I. For about 30 minutes we looked for John, enlisting the help of airport staff along the way. At last, Lisa and the girls found him calmly waiting for the rest of us at the new gate. He was smiling and glad to see that they "finally made it." Lisa called back to Bob and me that John was there! What a relief it was to know that he was there and that he was able to get himself there on his own steam. As Bob and I rushed to join them at the gate, it lifted my spirits and helped me to hold onto the hope that the confusion might still be just the aftermath of the seizure. Perhaps the seizure was caused by necrosis and the damage already done by the previous surgeries and treatment. While serious, this was certainly a better prospect than a second recurrence of the 2003 tumor.

Once we arrived at the Denver International Airport, we rented an SUV. It seemed strange not to have John's name at the head of the list of the drivers. He did not protest. He knew that he could no longer drive safely, and safety was his priority. He had no pretentious bone in his body and no false pride. He had always been a safe driver, never prone to impatience or speed behind the wheel. So now he accepted his limitations with dignity. On the trip to Estes Park, we stopped for dinner and all of us were in guarded, good spirits.

Well after dark we arrived at the YMCA camp, checked in and found our cabin in the woods. It was named the Broadview. We saw many curious deer in our headlights as we slowly made our way through the darkness to the cabin. In the morning, we awoke to a gorgeous "broad" view of the mountains. From our porch we could not see the other cabins in the area as they were located behind our cabin. It gave us a sense of being in a more remote wilderness area than it actually was. The deer and an occasional elk would venture across the pasture in front of us, and a trail could be taken across the meadow. The gravel roads behind us not only provided access to the cabins in this area, but were also another place for quiet walks. John was weak, and required a lot of rest. But he enjoyed brief walks by himself, and with me, the girls and Bob. Lisa watched from the porch. We all enjoyed feeding the birds on the rail of the cabin.

We had a little problem the first night. There were three bedrooms and two bathrooms. We agreed on the one that John and Lisa would take and the one that Bob and I would take. The "girls" logically would take the room with bunk beds and an additional single bed. But logic did not prevail when the girls started hearing noises in the wall behind their beds. We all assumed that there were rats in the wall. Mary Kaitlin and Carly would have none of it! John and Lisa traded rooms with them for the rest of the night. We considered moving to another available cabin the next day. After visiting it, we did not want to move. It did not have the beautiful location that the Broadview had. It was the same floor plan, but was not as recently updated with fresh paint and furnishings. Fortunately that afternoon, John discovered that our "rats" were really baby birds. After that it was much easier to co-exist with the scratching sounds in the bedroom wall. The girls eventually returned to their bunk beds and John and Lisa, to the room that they had before the "rat" scare.

The first full day of our visit, the girls started attending YMCA camping activities, and enjoying every minute of it. The rest of us busied ourselves bringing in groceries, bird seed, and exploring Estes Park by car. John especially wanted to go trout fishing. He had not brought his own fly rod, but there were rods to be rented at the YMCA headquarters, which we did. We purchased a fishing license for John and one for me. Then we packed a lunch and the four adults drove up to a mountain lake, well known for fishing opportunities. This place had an early history as a fishing retreat under private ownership. In its more recent history and up to the present, it is a part of the National Park. As luck would have it, it was very windy the day that we went to the lake. It was difficult to impossible to fly fish because of the wind. Tying flies was not easy either. John's left hand and arm were becoming weaker and more difficult to use, especially for an intricate task like fly tying. My arthritic fingers plus lack of prior experience tying flies ruled me out as a good helper. We ate our picnic lunch, enjoyed the beautiful mountain scenery, and returned to Broadview in time to greet the girls returning from camp. We had no fish but were armed with determination to try again.

The next day we drove to the top of the mountain pass (Trail Ridge Drive), while the girls were participating in their camping activities. John, Lisa, Bob and I enjoyed the trip. We saw snow and ice, lots of streams of melting snow, elk, chipmunks and marmots.

During the week, I enjoyed doing most of the cooking for the

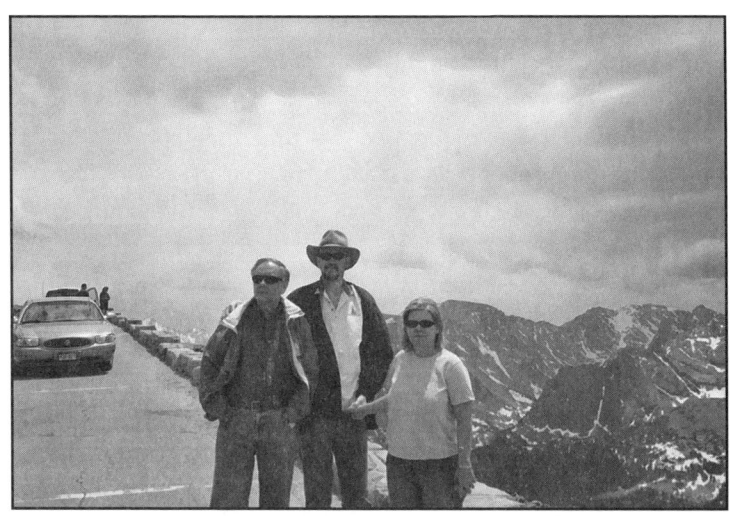

*John, Lisa and Bob posing for a picture
that I took on the mountain top of Trail Ridge Drive.*

family, giving Lisa as much opportunity to relax and rest as I could. We both participated in the grocery shopping and especially enjoyed the variety of fresh produce we found there. John rested most of the time when we were in the cabin. Sometimes he would get up and play with his beloved daughters. He took a pretty hard spill playing with Carly, but did not hit his head nor seem to be hurt in any way by it. An even less fortunate incident happened when he lost his balance sitting on the edge of his bed and fell into the bedside table, taking a hard hit on the back of his head. I examined it and could see that there was some redness there, but it subsided and did not leave swelling or a lump. It apparently did not create any more complications to the ones that he already had, but it hurt all of us for him to have suffered this unnecessary blow. Both of these incidents resulted from John's deteriorating condition, which was making him weaker and much less steady on his feet.

One night, Sally's mother and father-in-law Dot and Pete Jackson came to visit. Dot had been hiking with some of her lady friends from Boulder, where she and Pete live. The friends dropped her off at our cabin and Pete drove there. It was good to have them. John was holding up as best he could, and was glad to see them, but

I am sure that they were astounded at how gaunt and ill that he looked. The harsh chemotherapy and the cancer had taken an enormous toll.

Nevertheless, we all savored this time together. We built fires in our living room fireplace and went fishing the second time. We took frequent short walks with John and longer rides enjoying the wildlife and views.

One day as we sat in front of one of the YMCA camp buildings, we discovered our rental car's tire was flat. John was accustomed to changing tires and fixing things that were broken, so he wanted to fix the tire. I gently protested and he backed off reluctantly, as he realized that now it was beyond his strength and agility. The father of another family parked next to us, recognized our predicament and he graciously changed the tire. It was hard work as the parking area was gravel and not level. We watched him work, and I felt some envy along with my appreciation for his help. It seemed so unfair for John not to be strong, healthy and able like the husband and father who was helping us so kindly. Bob and I privately shared how "bitter sweet" our vacation felt. We had this awful feeling and awareness, that barring a miracle, this would possibly be the last summer that John would be with us. Hanging over us like a shadow was the fear of what we would learn when we returned home.

I remember so well an especially touching time for me when the six of us went to the town of Estes Park on a shopping trip. John and I had spotted a knife shop in the town center, which was of some considerable interest to John, since he collected knives. So after our car was parked, he and I decided to walk to the knife shop to take a look. We unknowingly took the long way around, walking hand in hand until we got there, both to steady John and to comfort each other as we walked, mostly in silence. In the shop, when I saw John about to buy a little inexpensive knife out of a basket, I encouraged him to look further. We left all smiles, with a "boot knife" for a late birthday present. It was a type of knife that he did not have in his collection and he was very pleased to have it.

A few days before leaving Colorado, we took John for one last attempt to catch a trout in a beautiful Colorado stream. We left him there alone for about an hour, to fish, to observe the beauty around

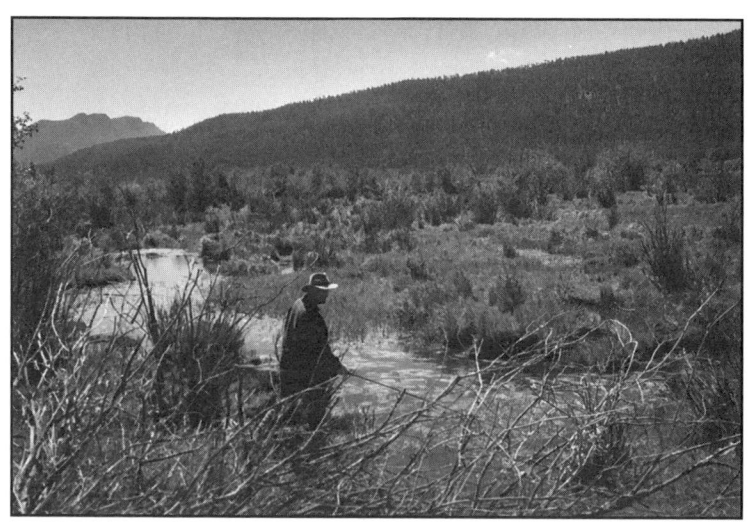
John as we found him when we returned to pick him up on the last day of fishing.

him and no doubt, to contemplate. On our return to the spot to pick him up, we found him still fishing, smiling and content though he had not caught a fish.

On the day of our departure, while driving back to the airport, we finally got the trout that eluded us in the Colorado streams. It was smoked trout, purchased in a shop that we had discovered on prior trips. We could take it back to Texas unrefrigerated and keep it in its sealed package for a long time. John enjoyed the smoked trout with friends from San Antonio, who came to see him later in the summer. As I write this in January of '05, I still have my smoked trout! Like with so many "things" that remind me of John, I do not want to give it up. Arriving home on Sunday, June 12, we were glad to have had the trip, but our hearts were heavy as we faced the next step, an MRI on Monday and an appointment with Dr. Groves on Tuesday.

On June 13, I wrote the following in my journal.
Today I am thankful for the trip that we have had with Lisa, John and the girls. We are safe at home, at least safe in the sense of our travels. The girls enjoyed their respective camp experiences, while the grownups enjoyed the weather, the beautiful scenery, and watching

elk, deer, coyotes, birds, wild flowers and the mountain tops – all from the view of our front porch, as well as several drives around the National Park on Trail Ridge Drive and other byways. John and Lisa's courage and love for each other and their girls are inspiring and beautiful to see. I am very proud of them as I watch them embrace life in the face of so much illness. I am frightened as we approach tomorrow and the MRI and Tuesday, when they will see Dr. Groves regarding the new MRI. John's impairment on the left side seems worse than 3 weeks ago. We pray and hope for an explanation other than cancer. Then I recorded the following scripture: *Answer me quickly, O Lord. My spirit fails. Do not hide your face from me or I shall go down into the pit. Let me hear of your steadfast love in the morning for in you I put my trust. Teach me the way I should go, for to you I lift up my soul.* **Psm. 143.7-8**

The radiologist report of June 14 revealed that the enhancements had significantly grown in the three weeks since the previous MRI. While the report provided good news pertaining to a small spot in the right frontal lobe that the doctor had been watching for several months, it was completely overshadowed by the bad news about the increased enhancements in the area of the resection cavity in the right inferior parietal lobe

Once again and for the third time in less than a year and one half, we turned to the possibility of surgery. Dr. Groves was cautious in the evaluation of the extent to which surgery might prolong his life at this point. The location of the "enhancement" was now even closer to the motor strip, impinging upon it, causing John to become weaker on the left side of his body. But with our support, John decided to have the surgery. More than anything, he wanted to stay with his wife and daughters as long as he could, even if it meant using a wheelchair. We assured him of how much we wanted him to remain with us, wheelchair included. He said; "I can live with the wheelchair." He was basing that assumption on the strong hope that the surgery would give him another chance to put the cancer into remission. In the same breath, he said; "It's not the wheel chair, it is the cancer that will get me."

Dr. Groves asked us to see Dr. Prabhu, a neurosurgeon in the Brain and Spine Center of MDA. He wanted us to stay inside the

MDA system this time so that if John did have the surgery, he could be treated comprehensively during his stay in the hospital. I described what we were going through as a result of the MRI and the appointment with Dr. Groves in my journaling of June 16.

We have been through two days of anxiety, hope, fear, agony. John's MRI shows further enhancement, but Dr. Groves still says that it looks like necrosis and given John's history of treatment that diagnosis makes sense. However, he said that there could be cancer combined with the necrosis. He said that we cannot know for sure without a biopsy, which John agreed to have. Then Dr. Groves will know and determine what to do in terms of further treatment. The good news is that hope remains, since Dr. Groves clearly plans to continue treatment. John still has a chance that this will be controlled. It is so hard to see my son have to go through this awful valley. I feel so helpless, sad, and wanting so much to be able to protect him and nurse him back to health. If I could only wave a magic wand and put myself in his place and free him to be well. Then I closed my journaling with a prayer.

Dear God, Be with John, Lisa and the girls, Watch over and take care of them. Give us all faith and belief in that which is unseen – that which you have promised. Help each one of us to do those things that we cannot possibly do, left to our own resources. I ended with the following scripture: *In the fear of the Lord one has strong confidence and one's children will have a refuge."* **Proverbs 14.26**

After the first visit to Dr. Prabhu, the final decision was made to have the biopsy. Dr. Prabhu also told us that because of the previous surgeries, a plastic surgeon would have to be involved in the surgery in order to close the wound. My June 21 journal entry reflects the agony that John and those who love him faced.

We anxiously wait for the biopsy – hoping, hoping. Sally and Will came down to be with John before going on their family trip to the Hudson River Valley in New York. They had an enjoyable and comforting visit with John. Will, Mary Kaitlin and Carly had fun together as always. All of us, including Rene, had dinner together on Thursday night. John has had a good appetite since going off of chemo. On Saturday, West came. He and John also got in some good time together – in addition, West replaced the girl's bathroom door which had been broken after Carly had locked herself in several months ago. The door was broken in an unsuccessful attempt to remove the door knob. John was too sick to repair the damage caused. West also shaved John and trimmed his beard. John looked so nice after that at church yesterday. Though his impairment on the left side continues to increase, much of his confusion and disorientation is gone. He is using his one temporary hearing aid that we got last Friday. Today, we returned to get the mold made for his right ear. After the audiology appointment, John wanted to eat at the Black Eyed Pea on Holcomb Street, as he recalled the two of us eating there 20-21 years ago, when he was first being treated for a brain tumor.

I continued with a prayer entry. *Lord, you are our rock – our redeemer. You lift us up with your loving presence when we could not possibly walk alone. You are John's refuge, his strength in times of trouble. Let me and all of his family, never tire of being a channel for your love for him. Amen*

My next journal entry was on June 22: *Bob invited Rev. Tom Pace to our house tonight for a healing service for John. John and Lisa wanted this very much and it went very well. John's friend from his Disciples Bible Study, Dan Ostrander, was there. John had previously dubbed him in his affectionate and whimsical way – "Disciple Dan." Rene was there as was Cheryl, who came today from Shreveport to help out with the girls while the rest of us were focused on John and his biopsy. There was much love and support for John expressed by all of us. Tom's scripture and words of faith, love and healing lifted our spirits one and all. John was comforted. Tom read from the Psalm 103, and from several passages in the NT – one from Mark about anointing with oil to heal.*

John had the biopsy at MDA on June 25. It revealed that he had highly active and malignant tumor cells combined with the necrosis next to the resection cavity involving the right inferior parietal lobe. Thus, our worst fears were confirmed that the substantial increase in enhancing tissue in relationship to the resection cavity involving the right inferior parietal lobe was not necrosis alone, but a deadly progression of the malignant disease. I noticed that the doctors were beginning to refer to the cancer as *Glioblastoma, Grade IV*. This term was now used reluctantly as the doctors could see a dramatic advancement of the speed that the cancer was spreading. We had been told at the very beginning in 1983 and again after the first biopsy and before the first surgery in 2003, that while the pathologist had graded his tumors as Astrocytoma III, there was a certain level of subjectivity in determining between grade III or IV – Astrocytoma III or Gliobastoma. Now after receiving the last MRI report and the preliminary pathologist report on the biopsy, we had to accept the fact that John's tumor, always classified as a fast growing glioma tumor, was growing faster than ever before. This news was devastating.

When I returned home that dark night I once again wrote in my journal the following notes.

After the biopsy, Dr. Groves discussed the surgery and its risks this time around. John, with the support of all of his family, confirmed their prebiopsy decision that they wanted to go for it. Dr. Groves told us that the Surgery was scheduled for July 2.

The events came rapidly in July. It was July 18 before I made the next entry in my journal just two weeks and two days after the surgery. Sadly, this was the third brain surgery in a year and four months. In my July 18 journal entry, I recapped the time from June 25 until July 18. I noted just about everything that had happened since my previous entry on June 21. These days were so traumatic and so painfully fresh in my memory. Yet throughout this time, John continued to hope, and like a tree with decaying roots embedded in the sharp incline of a cliff, his family clung desperately along with him to whatever hope that was left.

From the day of the biopsy to the day of surgery was just one week. In that short time, a second MRI revealed that the cancer had continued to spread rapidly. The doctors planned to keep John in the hospital between the two procedures, but he insisted on going home. Under pressure from John and with our support for John's wishes, the doctors decided to let him go home for Wednesday and Thursday night to be with his beloved Lisa and the girls. He had to go in a wheel chair confiscated from MDA, as he could no longer walk after the biopsy. His brother West lifted him in and out of the wheel chair making the trip home possible. The main reason that the doctors had not wanted him to leave the hospital between the biopsy and surgery was because of concern about his safety. We were not yet well prepared at home to care for him. Nor had he had the benefit of rehabilitation through physical and occupational therapy, which would follow the surgery, making it safer for him to go home.

Before dawn on Friday, June 23, we had to have him back at the hospital for his surgery. His father, stepmother and West were staying at his house so West and Lisa took him back to the hospital. Sally and I went directly to the hospital in time to be there when he left his waiting area for surgery. I rushed into the cubicle afraid that I would not get to tell him I loved him before he went into the operating room. When I entered, a doctor, with nurses helping, was screwing a huge steel contraption to his head that had to be positioned with absolute accuracy. They asked me to help, instructing John to fasten his gaze upon me and for both of us not to move. As John looked at me, I will never forget the courage and love that I saw in his brown eyes, set within such a handsome and youthful face, refreshed by a month and one half without chemotherapy. We could not pray out loud before he was wheeled away, as there was too much presurgery activity going on with the doctors and nurses in the cubicle. Our prayers were unspoken.

Then during surgery, our family regrouped. Bob came from his office to join those of us who had gone earlier. We all sat together through the agonizing hours in the waiting room. Sally comforted herself by drawing abstract images that would later be in a series of art exhibits in Dallas community colleges and galleries. They were a series of small drawings that she entitled simply "John's drawings."

As previously mentioned, a plastic surgeon had to be called in for the surgery because previous operations, radiation and chemotherapy resulted in not having enough viable skin to cover the wound. The plastic surgeon's work accomplished all of its objectives, and the surgical area was covered in healthier tissue and more thoroughly than it had been for some time. But bringing sadness beyond measure was the news from Dr. Prabhu, the neurosurgeon, that he had been able to remove only 90% of the tumor. We had been told prior to surgery that they needed to get about 98% of it to have the best chance of remission. That was not the worst news. Dr. Prabhu explained to us that what remained had grown into the ventricle and that part was inoperable. To surgically penetrate the ventricle would have led to instant death.

For the tumor to be in the ventricle had ominous implications for spread to other parts of the brain. John was told by us and the doctors that the surgery was not as successful as had been hoped, but to my knowledge no one told him about the ventricle. Nevertheless, at least a slim hope remained that the surgery plus a new round of chemotherapy would give him some time in remission. Therefore John was kept in the hospital past the week required for the surgery to sufficiently heal. He remained there until July 23, working with a team of occupational and physical therapist from the MDA Rehabilitation and Palliative Care Center to recover as much ability as possible. They even expressed hope that they might get him moving and problem solving with higher level thinking to the point that he could return to work. The plastic surgeon also seemed hopeful. He continued to monitor John's wound. He talked about how the wound was healing. He thought the wound would continue to heal although there were a few areas of concern, some ooze persisted and a dark area emerged where the skin had died. He thought that it would resolve itself since viable skin was probably underneath it. If not, he could correct it. His looking toward John's future and the improvement in the area of the wound again gave me faint hope, maybe the chemo would work at least for a while.

In the meantime I noted in my July 18 journal entry that we still did not know what his new chemotherapy would be since Dr. Groves was out of his office from the time of surgery until July 19. We were eager for John to start the chemotherapy, because we knew that the cancer was not necessarily waiting to begin its relentless march into other areas of the brain. While we were waiting, we used the time to have John's case reviewed at another major cancer center. We sent them John's MRI film, a medical history and proposed treatment. After their review, they told us that they had nothing to offer for John's advanced case other than the course of treatment that MDA was offering. Therefore we stayed the course with MDA.

Meanwhile, all of John's family pitched in to help during this time of crises – Blair and Charlotte, Sally, West, Rene, and in Baltimore, Tate and Kim. Sally took Mary Kaitlin and Carly to "summer camp" at her home "Camp Jackson" in Dallas for a week during John's lengthened stay in the hospitalization for rehab. Charlotte took care of the girls often, while Lisa would spend nights at the hospital. During John's stay from July 2 until July 23, he never spent a night alone, except the first two nights in ICU, where we were not allowed to stay. Those two nights had been a nightmare for John, literally and figuratively. If we could have stayed, it would have helped. After that either Lisa or I would take the night shift. Also, West stayed several nights and Sally stayed at least two nights, as I noted in my journal entry on July 18. Charlotte and Blair helped along with West to do many things that needed to be done to make Lisa and John's home environment safer and more convenient in anticipation of John's homecoming and most of all, to make it wheelchair accessible. This included West widening the door to the bathroom, Blair building a ramp for the back entry to the house and putting handicap rails in the water closet in the master bathroom. Sally bought a potty chair for John, and I bought a ramp for the side door of our house, so that his wheelchair could be rolled into our house for visits. At the end of my July 18 journal entry, a prayer reflects my continued hope. *Thank you God and please let John continue to improve and to have a good remission. Amen*

During the long hospital stay, John also wrote in his journal after Lisa brought it to him at his request. He made several entries although damage to his motor strip was now affecting his ability to write. Thus he printed in labored and brief entries as follows:

FRI - 7-9-04 HEARIADS (sic) TO BE READY. Underneath that note, he laboriously spelled correctly – HEARING AIDS. These were his second pair. The first set would not stay in place, so the second pair was ordered. They were made from the original molds, making it unnecessary for him to return to the audiologist's office. Therefore, I returned the first pair and picked up the second pair on Friday, July 9, as John's entry suggested and delivered them to him in the hospital. With his illness as advanced as it was, he never adapted to them very well, though he did wear them some and reported hearing better with them. He usually wore them for the physical and occupational therapy that began while he was in the hospital, as all of his therapists encouraged him to do. We hoped that a trip back to the audiologist for adjustments would help, but he was never again well enough to go.

John made additional entries on July 15, 22, and 23. His July 15 entry was longer and sadder than the other three. It reflects that John was in pain and he must have been frightened by all that was happening to him. He was feeling very anxious and eager to get back home. Yet, he wanted to do everything that he could to cooperate with his medical treatment, physical therapy and occupational therapy that were being provided while he was in the hospital. The doctors told him that they did not want him to go home until it would be safe for him. Their goals were to teach him how to transfer safely to his wheel chair and to maneuver around the house as much as possible with the aid of a "Heimie"walker.

In his July 15 entry, John used upper and lower case printing appropriately, spelled almost everything correctly. His quality of his printing and verbiage showed a good bit of improvement over the entry of July 9. This was apparently due to reduced swelling and the healing that was taking place at the surgical site. I have typed his entry exactly as he wrote it.

JULY 15, 04: *"Injured heel when left leg free fell yesterday from elevated rest. Free fell into good foot and free fel (sic) hard floor, bruised left heel.*
Wed. focal seizure in face, not getting prescribed amount of Dilantin: Dilantin level 4.7
Skin graft area is still weeping clear fluid, still cannot reliably get from wheelchair to bed w/o assistance from staff.
Left arm leg and hand severely weakend (sic) by surgery.

Then his last two brief entries follow:
7 - 22: *Started chemo last night*
7 - 23: *discharged from Hospital*

Chapter 5

GOING HOME

"Most of all, I want you both to know I would never leave you."

John was so glad to get home. He continued to fight hard to live during the next six weeks, after his discharge from the hospital. While he said repeatedly that he was "not afraid to die" and meant it, he wanted so much to live in order to be there to give love to his family and all that he could give them in the way of material and spiritual support. He tried so hard not to leave them. He was sent home with a chemotherapy protocol that included CCNU, which he had taken for the year following his first brain tumor surgery in 1983. This time, Celebrex was also given in hopes that it would work to make the CCNU more effective.

During the month of August, while taking the chemo, John continued physical and occupational therapy at MDA. I drove him there from Sugar Land and stayed with him, until time to return home. For the first two weeks of August, he made some progress. He learned how to improve his balance so that he did not lean so far to the right as he was prone to do as a result of the damage to his motor strip. He also learned to "walk" on the parallel bars, carefully putting his right foot forward and then dragging his left foot up to the right foot. This was preparation for the way he would be instructed to walk with the aid of a one- sided Heimie walker. He pedaled a stationery bicycle that was designed so that his wheelchair could be pulled up to it allowing him to continue to sit in it while pedaling. His occupational therapist, Marguerite, encouraged him to do something that he enjoyed doing. As a result, he brought his spinning rod to therapy, and with Marguerite and me at his side, he tried casting on the lawn of MD Anderson. The day that he tried this, it was hot and humid as only August in Houston can be. He was weak and the lawn casting did not work so well, but it did bring some smiles and faint hope to John as he attempted it. A bitter sweet breath of hope came to me too, as I watched his effort.

John and all of his family held on to hope for improvement and remission as long as we could. Using the Heimie walker on Wednesday of the second week of his out patient physical therapy, he actually walked for 130 feet as measured by Marco, his therapist that day. We were encouraged. The goal was for John to be able to use the walker as an adjunct to the wheel chair in order to get around the house with it in a limited way. Perhaps he could reach the goal!

But by the middle of August, John could feel himself slipping further toward death. The very next day after he walked with the Heimie walker for 130 feet around the rehab facility, he could manage to walk only a few steps. At home, he told me that he believed that many tumors had spread all over his brain. I helplessly and ineptly responded that I thought it was probably just one, though possibly growing, thinking somehow that that was a more hopeful explanation. I was trying to offer comfort, but in retrospect, I know that response could not have been any comfort to him. It would have been better had I just held his hand or perhaps asked him if he felt like telling me more about what he was experiencing.

John's next scheduled MRI was not until August 30. Knowing that his cancer was spreading, he did not want to wait so long for the MRI. He was convinced that the chemotherapy was not working. He asked me; "Why are the doctors so rigid?" My response was to get him an early appointment at about 4 weeks into the chemo cycle with Dr. Groves. At the appointment, Dr. Groves explained to him that an early MRI could be done, but he did not encourage it. He said that it was possible that the chemo would begin to work in the last two weeks of the six-week cycle, because the CCNU, which had been taken orally for the first four weeks, would still be in his system. Also because of the CCNU still being in his system, he could not begin a new treatment until after the six weeks cycle was over. Therefore John agreed with the doctor to wait and hope against hope. We had no place else to turn for medical help. However, our church community and neighbors continued to be of help. Much food was brought to the house during this time. Lisa and all of us were spared planning meals and cooking them for the most part. Men friends that John had made during his Disciple's bible study and other church activities, set up a schedule to alternate visits with John. His fellow employees at

Weston called, visited and kept him as full time employee throughout his entire ordeal. His closest friends from San Antonio came to Sugar Land several times – Ashby and Joanie, Reb and Barb and Gary and Andrea. They laughed, cried and comforted John, recalling good times from the past.

Some days, we would take John outside on the back terrace where he had a vantage point from which he could watch his dogs, hummingbirds, redbirds and others that would come to a bird feeder strategically placed. Sally and I took him for outdoor walks, pushing his wheel chair along the sidewalk and around a few blocks. The heat was fierce, but the shaded sidewalks helped as well as the fact that John at this point in the illness tended to feel cold even in the heat. Lisa was with him day and night, reassuring him with her love, listening to his prayers, concerns and wishes, being as West said – his angel.

During this time of obvious and rapid tumor growth as manifested by John's continued decline, and increasing paralysis, there were many tears, his and ours. The left side of his body was now almost completely paralyzed. The right side was getting weaker, but he was not paralyzed on the right side. His right sided smile attested to his indomitable and loving spirit. The ability still remaining on his

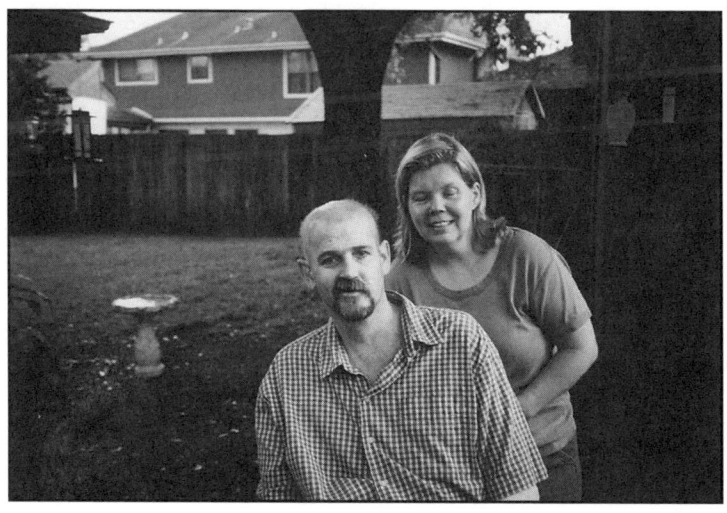

John in his wheelchair with Lisa in their back yard, August, 2004.

right side, though limited, was enough for him to speak, pray and laboriously write letters to his wife, children, and other family members. His faltering handwriting reflected the continued progression of the tumor, but more important are the messages that he wrote, which convey his selfless and abiding love for his Maker and for all of his family.

<u>John's Letters (August 18 - 29, 2004)</u>

August 18, 2004
(John to his daughters Mary Kaitlin and Carla Jane)
Dear - my blessed children. I love you so much. The hand of Jesus is not in this disease - you are both so talented and smart. Please don't let my passing hurt your faith in the Lord. God's hand is only in good. He has brought me much comfort in these days. I am so glad you will continue.

I love your mother and through her, we will be connected always. I love you beyond measure. I am so happy that you will be living with your mother. She will need lots of love that I know you two will provide. I am so sorry I won't be there.
I will always love you both,
Daddy

Most of all I want you both to know I would never leave you.

August 20, 2004
Dear Precious Family,
I love you. I'm sorry that I'm being called away. All that I have been living for is to watch you grow up. I have forgotten a lot of things. I do know that I was always loved by my family. I'm sorry you had to endure this. I love you all very much. I pray for the best things in life for all of you.

August 21, 2004
John to Lisa
I have prepared to die so many times. I don't want to for the sake of my children. Let me watch my children grow and see what they become. I love you.

John to Lisa
You can be sure that every night I pray for another night with you. Tell them that my love is unconditional. Love, Daddy

August 21, 2004
Sally
I have always loved you. You have been a protector and provider for me and my family. As good as you are, you and Jeff raised fine children, filled with aspirations and kindness. I love you much, Sister.

I want you and my family to mourn and cry as much as you need. I wish God's blessings and then go on with what you have been doing.

I trust you to help my children emotionally to get them thru this – holding siblings together – explain always together, talking your way thru.

Then John was tiring and asked Sally to write the following for him; I know it's hard to read, but between the 3 entries, it should not be too hard to figure out.

August 21, 2004
John to West
Brother West,
You endured while I was a pest. I have idolized you for as long as I can remember, Brother West. I have loved and idolized you since you helped me to grow up, not by giving me the perfect example but by showing me what works and what does not in relationships. I have always loved you even in the middle of pretzel holds. It is fair to say (to) you, I still idolize your strength and abilities (lifting me?) And drive to accomplish.

John to Mother
Cry as long as you need to then join/let your family and friends support you. You have been a wonderful, superb mother and I could not have asked for a better mom. I love you,
Your loving son,
John
And please live life to the fullest, you deserve it. I love you so much,
John

While John was writing letters, Sally also wrote a letter to him. I did too.

8/23/04
Sally to John
Dear John,
You have been working each day to write letters to your family, telling them how much they mean to you, and trying to give them something of yourself to hold onto. So I want to send you a letter to hold onto, in the form of a few memories and thoughts.

Do you know how important you are?

I actually remember the day you came home from the hospital–I was 5 and got to climb up on your crib rail, set up in the big pink bedroom on Burnside. As older sister, I felt that you were my personal baby doll, as well as that I was your self-appointed protector.

After a while, you and West became a glued-at-the-hip duo, and the two of you went your own ways, going about the business of being boys with all that meant. But I was still your protector when I thought you needed it.

And sometimes maybe you protected me. Did you know that after we moved to Huntleigh Lane, I would crawl into the antique bed with you at night when I was afraid? You were the peaceful brother, and I knew you would let me stay, and I would instantly feel better.

As you and I have talked about many times, we grew up and I had to make my own way apart from "the boys", and I think that especially in high school and college our age difference separated us too.

But as we became adults, I missed my little brother, and we started to be friends again. We could talk. You were there for me even though I don't know if you knew it. You came to see me in New York before I married Jeff. That meant a lot.

I was a newlywed living in Chicago when you became sick the first time, and I think I was drawn back into our family by the need to pull together for you. I am sure that's why Jeff and I moved back to Dallas, from the distress of that experience and being so far away. You came to see me in Chicago, too, after your cancer treatments.

We have had 20 years of miracle since then, with no one taking your life for granted, except maybe you, since you had to live it and go about the blessed ordinariness of daily family life. Your happy marriage is a miracle, your children are a miracle, and your faithful and loving participation and enjoyment of your family has been glue which binds us all together. You are so important.

Perhaps from the suffering you have had in your own life, you have a generosity of spirit which lets you forgive and overlook disappointments and appreciate the good in others. You're just naturally sweet, as Bea used to say, funny too. And did I mention handsome?

Right now you are grieving, exhausted from the effort to cope with the paralysis, and trying to say and do the right things for your family. You are feeling spiritually disconnected from God, and not knowing where to find hope. I think there are ways to find hope which God provides, which we don't usually consider. We hope for a cure, or we hope for an afterlife which maybe sort of resembles what we love about this life. Those are good hopes and major ones, but I think God provides some smaller hopes that are important too.

There is hope in the beautiful order of nature, where the mystery of God's law is laid out for us to see as clearly as if it was written in the sky. In nature God says this:
There is a plan. There is a reason for things to happen. Everything is connected.
Life endures. Nothing is lost.

There is hope in the resolution of unfinished business. By reaching out to all of your family, by making sure that your girls know you are thinking of them and know what you are thinking, you are acting to make sure that your concern and love for them will carry on forever, no matter what happens. And you are giving yourself a means of peace.

There is hope in the enjoyment of any small moment of your day, because surely enjoyment is a major gift of life, and something to be so grateful for. This weekend I enjoyed being with you in spite of all the pain, because there were moments when the pain loosened its grip a little, such as when we went for a walk, or when you sang along with the Flintstones and Jetsons songs on the piano. (I knew you would since you have that talent for singing.) And that reminds me I have always enjoyed your basic drollery and tom-foolery, including your comment this weekend about the fluffy bunny tail (ask Lisa) which still makes me laugh.

So my hope for you this week is this: Try to enjoy some small and specific things about the girls, Lisa, life. Sing some more silly songs. Enjoy the breeze. You are important.

Your loving sister,
Sally

Mother to John
8/28/04
My dearest John,
I want to thank you for telling me so many times and then writing to me lately, to tell me how much I mean to you as your mom. I have told you too, how much you mean to me. But now, I want to write it down for you as well – just how dearly and deeply that I love you, and how proud I am of you now and how proud I have always been of you, my precious son.

You have always been such a good son to me, and I have watched proudly as you have gone about your life, being such a loving and devoted husband to Lisa and father to Mary Kaitlin and Carly. Before that, I watched you grow up so sweet and gentle, treasuring and building loving relationships with me, your grandparents, father, brother, sister, and friends, then Papa Bob, Rene, Kim and Scott as well. You handled your first bout with cancer at such a young age with courage beyond your years. I am so proud of your finishing at A&M under such difficult circumstances and then I am proud of all of the hard work that you have done through the last approximately 18 years as an environmental engineering consultant. The way the men and women of Weston have rallied around you during the last 18 months is testimony to your character and work ethic. You have been a good and humble servant of our Lord from childhood, active in your churches in San

Antonio, College Station, and here in Sugar Land. With Lisa, you set the example for your girls to lead good lives filled with faith in God through His Son and you continue to encourage them in every way. Each place and heart that you have touched you have left better than you found it and you continue to do so each day of your life. Our faith confirms for us that those who love each other as we do, can never really be separated for love, like life, is Eternal – a gift from our Heavenly Father. We abide in Him now and we will for evermore.

I love you with all of my heart and soul now and forever,

Mother

John also used prayer as a constant source of comfort, communicating both to God and to his family through his prayers. He would pray out loud while either Lisa or I, or both of us, were with him. I realized how much I would like to have recorded those prayers, so on one occasion I made mental notes as he prayed, and then wrote as much down as I could remember immediately after he finished. Here are my notes recalling much of this prayer.

*Father, I have not been your greatest servant, but I love you. Forgive me. Bless all of my family, Lisa, Mary Kaitlin, Carly, Sally, West, my father, my mother, and all of the rest of my family. John then added a supplication especially for his wife and mother, recognizing in his prayer that they would be heart broken. He asked that God help them grieve and then to move on with their lives. John then thanked God for Mary Kaitlin and Carly, and thanked God that they have such a good mother to look after them. As he continued, he asked God to let him "be the **lamb**," to suffer this disease and to never let his children or anyone else in his family become its victims. He prayed that what the doctors learned from his experience would help others afflicted with this disease. He prayed for relationships within the family to be strong and in his extended family to be healed where there was hurt. Then he quoted from the 23rd Psalm; "Yea though I walk through the valley of death, I will fear no evil." Again he gave thanks for his life, his wife and children.*
Amen

Chapter 6

PLAN D

"Mother is hard to refuse!"

The six weeks of the first cycle of CCNU was over in the third week of August and John once again had an MRI. As was standard procedure, the next day John, Lisa, Bob and I went to see Dr. Groves. Dr. Groves told us what John had verbalized and what the rest of us already knew in our hearts. The cancer was spreading out of control. Dr. Groves told John "to get his affairs" in order. Then he corrected himself to say that he knew that John had no doubt already done this. It was only on this visit that Dr. Groves realized that John had two daughters that he would leave behind.

Courageously and with his dry wit battered but still intact, John would not give up and so he asked; "Well doctor, what is Plan D?" He was referring to the fact that he had now exhausted three protocols – Plans A, B, and C, which included three surgeries, each followed by a different chemotherapy. Dr. Groves' distress, as for the rest of us, was palpable on this occasion, but he offered no Plan D. John cried and tears were quietly flowing everywhere in the examining room. As we sat there stunned, I plowed my distraught mind to think of some other chemotherapy that I had read about on the internet. I came up with Accutane, and I asked Dr. Groves if perhaps John could try that. He responded that he did not think that it would hurt John, and added weakly that it had occasionally helped someone. So Accutane, a medication originally developed for treatment of acne, was prescribed to be given orally each day. It hardly seemed like a Plan D, but apparently it was the best that MDA could do at this point in time. Therefore, I took to the internet, once again to look for alternatives.

I was particularly interested when I found information on the internet about the Burzynski method of treatment. When I found this, I recalled that years before I had read in our newspapers about a controversy over treatment that Dr. Burzynski was using for treating brain tumors. At that time, though John was well, I had taken special interest in it because of the medical history of his first brain tumor. Those old newspaper reports had indicated that Dr. Burzynski was having trouble with the FDA and with a skeptical medical community. But the news reports also indicated that his patients defended him, as many believed he had helped or cured them. This had caught my attention because, even though I had become more confident over the years that John would never be faced with a brain tumor again, there always remained in my mind a level of concern and anxiety that it could happen. Then in April of 2004 when John was 5 months into Plan B (the Cisplatin chemotherapy) that followed his second surgery within a year, I heard again about Dr. Burzynski. This happened while I was attending a luncheon where I had a conversation with an acquaintance of mine. Knowing of John's battle with brain cancer, she told me about the Burzynski Clinic and its successes, some of which she knew about personally. She urged me to consider it. This was just one month before the May MRI, which resulted in John's removal from Cisplatin protocol, followed by his third surgery in July and subsequently, the CCNU. And now in early September of 2004, MDA had no more treatment alternatives for a patient with his history and stage of cancer, but I simply could not give up trying to find something to save John from imminent death within the next six weeks to 3 months according to Dr. Groves's predictions.

Sometimes miracles happen. For the last twenty one years, John had been among those counted as a miracle! Even now, seven months after John's death, I see a "miracle" reported on the front page of the Houston Chronicle. Here is what the Houston Chronical reports (May 26, 2005); "Advanced skin cancer patient J. Newman was getting his final affairs in order last year when he began a Houston trial (at MDA) of an experimental new treatment." Then the article goes on to say that Mr. Newman's melanoma had resisted surgery and chemotherapy and spread to his lungs in tumors too numerous to count. But now he was back to his old self, working in his shop, building things, playing golf. This was the kind of possibility or miracle upon which my mind and heart were set, so I initiated contact with the Burzynski Clinic. As John had already said, he too wanted another chance, surely more so than I or any of the rest of his loved ones could even imagine. Thus I contacted the Burzynski Clinic, and they were receptive to seeing him.

On September 9, John, Blair, Lisa and I went to the Burzynski Clinic where Dr. Gabor Jurida conducted an extensive interview while referring to copious records and images that we had previously brought to the clinic, records that went back to John's treatment from 1983 until the present. We were impressed by the doctor's thoroughness. At the end of the rather long day at the clinic, he determined that they would treat John within the parameters of their investigational clinical study that had been approved by the FDA. To make it official, John initialed a "Statement of Informed Consent for Investigational Clinical Study," which was a Phase II study of antineoplastons A10 and AS-1. The consent gave detailed information about the treatment as previously discussed that day. We were informed that these antineoplastons are chemically converted in solution to phenylacetic acid and to phenylacetylglutamine, a compound formed in the body when phenylacetic acid is administered. The consent form stated that the phenylacetic acid is a material that slows the growth rate of some cancer cell types that are exposed to it in the test tube. The patient is advised of the protocol, the need for a catheter to permit administration of the treatment if one is not already in place, the training requirements for family members and the monthly physical examinations and laboratory tests that are required by the study protocol. Of course, possible risks were also enumerated. There were many, including central nervous system toxicity, decreased white blood cell count and liver toxicity all of which have serious affects, many of which John already exhibited, such as slurred speech, headaches, tiredness, and others. In extreme cases as with all previous consent forms required for John's treatments, we were advised that the treatment could result in death. John shook hands with Dr. Jurida, gave him a smile, and initialed the pages of the consent form with **JW**, written in a strong and clear script. John and the rest of us were also advised that he was being taken into the study as a "Special Exception" because his Astrocytoma III was at such an advanced stage that he did not qualify without the exception. In spite of the extremely dire condition that John was in, I perceived that he, Blair and I were visibly more "upbeat" when we left the clinic than we had been for a while.

The treatment planned was basically the same as I had read about many years before in the local newspaper and the one that my friend had recommended at the luncheon attended in May. It is the one that Dr. Burzynski had been using for many years at his clinic, but to date he did not have FDA approval to sell the medication Therefore insurance coverage was limited. The FDA study that John was to enter would hopefully lead to the medication being FDA approved.

Before leaving the clinic that day, Blair and I made it "official" by paying equally into a deposit, which was the amount of the first 6 weeks of treatment assuming no insurance coverage. Subsequently the account would be credited for some clinical services that were covered by insurance. When we returned home, John began drinking large amounts of water as prescribed for the pending treatment, as near to one gallon of distilled water per day as he could. He needed to work up to as close to two gallons a day as he could get by the time the treatment started.

The next day, September 10, we took John to an imaging center where he had an MRI and PET scan which were required by the protocol, prior to treatment. I remember that Blair, Sally, Lisa, and I took John that day. Sally had flown in the day before. She had not gone to the clinic for the initial visit with us and wanted to be with John and to see the clinic. John and all of us were very stressed as we waited while John once again had the MRI. John had had so many MRI's before and he tolerated them very well. But his desperate condition was the source of profound sadness with little to hope for as he faced the imaging and also a PET scan that day. To my knowledge this was the first time ever that a PET scan had been ordered for him. After the MRI and PET, Sally, Lisa and I delivered the images to Burzynski Clinic, while Blair took John home. Both Sally and Lisa were increasingly concerned about the wisdom of John's participation in the treatment program. Visiting the clinic for the first time, Sally was not relieved of her concerns. In the meantime, John had stopped the Accutane as required by the new protocol. Now all that was left was to wait until the Clinic had an appointment scheduled for insertion of a catheter, but as of September 13, that appointment was still pending. While waiting for the catheter over the weekend, we had a family gathering to discuss again whether or not we should put John through the treatment on the outside chance that the tumor might respond and shrink. I was frightened as we all were over the prospects of putting John through additional suffering that would not improve his condition. Therefore I agreed with the rest of us to withdraw John from the program and also agreed to be the one to tell him that we thought that it would be too much for him to endure. It was a very sad moment for all of us, but John with courage and dignity concurred. Instead of the new treatment we would start home health care, resume the Accutane, and try to keep John as comfortable as possible.

Then the next week, there was a news release on local television and across the state that the Burzynski antineoplastons were being put on a "fast track" for approval by the FDA. Lisa and I heard it together. After that, I became insistent that we reinstate John and give it a try. Lisa and Sally did not want him to be reinstated for the same reasons as before. They did not think it was possible for it to help and they wanted John to have a more peaceful quality of life as the end came. John agreed to try again, probably with greater reluctance than I realized at the time, as he later said; "Mother is hard to refuse." But to me, it was the only chance for a Plan D, and I could not let go of the slim hope that it would help him. Blair, Bob and West supported my position, but not without misgivings I am sure. Even I, with all of my denial, had misgivings.

We officially reinstated John on Monday, September 20. His appointment to insert the catheter was scheduled for Tuesday, September 21, and the clinical trial at the Burzynski Clinic was begun on Wednesday, September 22. Blair and I agreed to be John's caregivers throughout his treatment program. Blair's long term plan was to come from San Antonio to relieve me on a periodic basis. So he and I were required to take John to the clinic to learn how to administer the medicine on an ongoing basis. On the first day, John was given a thorough physical examination. I was impressed that from his wheelchair, John could still read the eye chart with complete accuracy. He had been blessed throughout his life with keen eyesight.

On Wednesday, John's nurse began teaching Blair and me what we would have to know to administer the treatment. We were given preliminary instructions on how to take care of the bags of medicine that had to be infused on a regular schedule of increasing dosages. We were also acquainted with the routine of using an automatic infusion pump. On Thursday, September 23, we were given more in-depth training on the care and maintenance of the infusion pump apparatus and the bags of medicine, as well as how to program the system for the proper dosages each day. Also, John was given a small trial dose of the medication by infusion at the clinic that day to make sure there was no allergic reaction. He tolerated it well.

But the next day, Friday September 24, things did not go well. We had a very long stay at the clinic. During the morning, most of the time was spent with the nurse teaching Blair and me more about how to take care of the bags of medicine to insure that no bubbles would be left in the bags once infusion began. Also, we were given more hands-on training about how to change the bags, how to work the digital controls to insure the proper dosage (which would increase over time), how to set the time for infusions to begin, and how to keep records on intake of water and output of urine. John waited patiently in his wheelchair. Though we could lower the back of the chair or raise it in attempts to make him more comfortable, he was not comfortable. He became extremely tired as the morning progressed. In the afternoon, John was left in the care of the nurse, while Blair and I were taken to the office of the clinic's nutritionist for instructions regarding John's diet and water intake. At that point, I think we both were feeling some hope, because the nutritionist was an optimistic person and knew what to tell us to do in terms of water intake and nutrition that would help prevent complications from the chemotherapy that would be infused into John's system.

In the meantime, the first bag of John's first daily dose of antineoplastons was attached to the pump and the infusion was started. Otherwise he continued waiting to go home, increasingly fatigued, but still trying to take liquids and to rest as best he could in his adjustable wheel chair with its tall back in a reclining position and a "table" that slid onto the arms of the chair to hold his snacks and drinks and to rest his arms.

The afternoon was wearing on when the last thing Blair and I were required to do was to go to the radiologist office in the clinic to see the PET scan and MRI that were done on September 10, as a prerequisite to this treatment. We were astonished at what we saw and were told. The cancer and the necrosis were everywhere on the right side of his brain. It was beginning to invade the left side, although ironically, the area of the frontal lobe at the site of John's first tumor was the least impacted. In addition to the cancer and necrosis, the right side of John's brain was virtually inundated with fluid. To me, the images looked more like those of rivers spilling over their banks than images of John's brain. The radiologist reviewing this with us did not give us much hope. We asked if John should be withdrawn from the treatment. His response was noncommittal, leaving that question for Dr. Jurida.

    John was more and more exhausted as the afternoon dragged on. His only relief from sitting or reclining in his wheel chair throughout the day had been a trip to the bathroom and a transfer to the toilet with Blair and me helping him. It was approaching 5:00 pm. Finally we could leave the clinic. When we got to the car and were figuring out how to transfer John without disconnecting or in any other way disrupting the flow of fluid into his body, we discovered that the infusion pump had been turned off. So anxiously, I called back to the nurse on my cell phone. She instructed us to simply push the button on the pump and the process would begin again. After that, we were successful in restarting the pump and in getting John transferred to the car. However the transfer had never been as hard as it was this time, because John had never been as weak as this. When we arrived home, because of his profound weakness and the lines of the connected pump, we once again had a very difficult time moving John from the car to his wheelchair and then to his bed. Blair, with help from a next door neighbor, was finally able to get him out of the car, into the house and then lift him to the proper position in his bed. Not long after he was situated in his bed for the night, he vomited small amounts of clear liquid twice.

    Seeing how weak, sick, and tired John was after the long day at the clinic, Lisa knew that John could not benefit from the new treatment. She wanted the quality of time that he had left to be better. So she talked to me again, asking me if I would be willing to forego anymore treatment. I agreed that I did not want him to suffer more, admitting that my hope was fading. I was beginning to see with the rest of our family that John was too sick to have any reasonable or even remote expectation that the treatment could help him get better. As evening approached, he was very tired and suffering from nausea and headaches. As the first bag emptied, the time was nearing to change bags in order to continue the infusion to completion of the first 24 hour dosage of two bags. He was weak and exhausted from the trip to the clinic and the new chemotherapy being administered, but mostly from the relentless progression of the cancer that had been taking him down in the last few weeks faster than we could have ever imagined.

In John and Lisa's bedroom, Lisa and John with their pastor Tom Pace at their side, made the decision not to proceed. The rest of us, Blair, Charlotte, Bob, Sally, West, Rene and I waited in the family room to be told. For me, it was the hardest moment of my life up until then, to bring myself to accept the truth that nothing more could be done to save John's life. But along with the rest of our family, I knew that it was true and so I supported the decision as the pump, our last hope, was detached and removed. Our hearts were breaking. All of us cried a lot that night.

We advised the Burzinski Clinic of our decision immediately after it was made on Friday night. Blair and I returned the pump and medicine on Saturday. Dr. Jurida met with us. He, the nurse who had cared for John, and other clinic staff were genuinely sad and disappointed, though understanding, when hearing of our decision. Dr. Jurida gave Lisa her initial instructions regarding John's Decadron dosages. We were to increase it gradually from 6 milligrams to 8 and then to 10 by Tuesday in order to better control brain swelling and thus headaches and seizures. John began doing a little better as a result of that in the brief interim before Hospice care began.

John had been receiving periodic home health care for about two weeks at that time. Now, Lisa immediately began making arrangements for Houston Hospice to provide John's care. Hospice will not come in until the family agrees to receive nothing other than palliative care, which precludes chemotherapy. The very next day, Saturday, September 25, a Hospice nurse came to evaluate and to get the process started. From then on, Hospice nurses, doctors, and social workers gave John and his family compassionate personal care as well as the medications that he needed to stay as comfortable as possible, mainly steroids and pain medication. A hospital bed was ordered and quickly delivered on Monday. Now John's paralysis and weakness made it completely impossible for him to get out of bed, so the hospital bed was critical to keeping him comfortable and free of bed sores.

On Tuesday September 28, I took Nerie to see him. She has been our housekeeper for over 20 years and had known John since before he had his first brain tumor. She is from Honduras and her first language is Spanish. Although I had tried to warn her, Nerie did not realize how sick John had gotten until she saw him that day, bed ridden and unable to move his extremities, except for limited movement in his right arm and leg. Upon seeing him, her tears came and she immediately began praying for him and consoling him in Spanish. As sick as he was, John still reciprocated and weakly spoke back to her in Spanish. He had taken Spanish in high school and college. Then he became more conversant using it while working in the West Texas oil fields during the semester that he took away from his studies between attending the University of Texas and his enrollment at A&M.

During Nerie's visit, I brought John potato soup. It was canned and he did not like it. He said; "Mother, no quiero." I coaxed him a little more to try it again. With a little grin on his face, he emphatically repeated; "Mother, no quiero papas!" Of course I gave up on the soup, but a little of his special humor was coming through. I think that he was enjoying the fact that he could still remember his Spanish when he rejected my offer. Afterward, Lisa told me, that when I was out of his room, that John started talking in Spanish to her. She reminded John that she could not understand him as she did not speak Spanish, to which he replied; "Go get Mother!" Again, I think that John was happy that he could remember his Spanish and he wanted to keep using it! Memory had become a constant worry for him. He was very aware and sad that he was having difficulty remembering things. This was particularly true of his short term memory, but he also complained that he was experiencing long term memory deficits.

While Nerie was still there, a group of his co-workers from Weston came to see him. Family left the room to make way for his colleagues, so that they could have a good visit with John. While they talked, we heard laughter and assumed things were going pretty well and that John was enjoying the visit. In retrospect, the visit was too long and exhausted him. It may have precipitated John falling into a steroid induced paranoid delusional state that afternoon, which lasted through the night and all of the next day and night. With this development, the lack of sleep and the emotional drain took its toll on John, and also the rest of us. Lisa contacted the Hospice nurse who instructed her to reduce the steroids from ten to eight and then to six milligrams, the level that would be continued until his death. With the steroids continued, John did not have more seizures but did continue to have some headaches. The headache pain was controlled by small morphine doses given in drops placed inside his cheek.

During the difficult delusional period, John continued to trust me and Lisa. He gave me instructions as to what to do to help prevent the catastrophic situations that he imagined were happening to his family, particularly his beloved daughters, who he wanted to protect so much. On minor things, I would go along with him, because I knew that this was caused by the tumor and its treatment with steroid and was not going to be alleviated by reason. On the major issues, such as thinking his daughters had died from toxic pollution to which he thought he had exposed them, or that lawyers were out to take everything he had away from his family, I would try to reassure him. I insisted that there were no such things, his daughters were fine and as for lawyers, they could not hurt him as he was the "good guy" who worked to clean up the environment, not to pollute it! I told him that Mary Kaitlin and Carly were at school, and would be home to see him soon. At one point when I was trying to reason with him, he looked at me with loving exasperation, and said; "Mother, you are *dopey*!" Even though I was dopey (I will not argue that point), he trusted me and gave me as well as Lisa "orders" as to what to do to protect his children from the danger of pollution or other perils.

After one sleepless day and two sleepless nights, Hospice prescribed Ativan. After taking his first and only dose, John slept all night and through the next day and night. The nurses told us that the Ativan was not why he slept for so long, but it was his weakness and deteriorating condition. I was afraid that he would not wake up.

But by Saturday, Oct 2, John woke up. He was calm and lucid, speaking to us, and recognizing his family and friends. At this time, Sally returned from Dallas. She was surprised that he recognized her and could smile and say a few things to her. He would occasionally say a few words and give each of us a one sided smile, one sided because of the paralysis on the left side of his face, which had grown increasingly more pronounced since his July surgery. One of many poignant moments after John rallied was when his lifelong friend "Reb" was there with his wife Barb from San Antonio. Reb and Barb helped in so many ways during those last two difficult weeks. This time Reb, Lisa, Sally and I were all in with John. Reb was observing John's "women folk" all trying to help him. Much to John's consternation, we were trying to gently move his neck to a new, more comfortable position as it was very stiff and had become a major source of pain as he lay bedridden. As John grimaced, Reb said with gentle humor, "John you've got to keep in mind that Lisa, Sally and Sara Jane are all "amateurs" so give them a little slack!" Through his pain, John responded with that knowing smile that was so special and his alone to give. Sally, Lisa and I all soothed John and tried to help him with his neck, but Barb, who is a licensed physical therapist worked magic with her hands, easing John's neck pain considerably on many occasions during the days when she and Reb were there.

As John's condition worsened, friends, neighbors and our church community seemed to never tire of caring for John. Food came almost daily. Prayers and visits were scheduled on a regular basis. His family was there for him – all of us.

Even those whose own burdens were almost too much to bear were there for him. John and Lisa's neighbor, Beth Van Sickle at 39 years of age was courageously battling metastasized breast cancer all of the while that John was fighting his battle. Lisa and Beth were friends and fellow warriors. As John's condition worsened, Beth and her husband Randy found many ways to help John and Lisa, often bringing food and in other ways they would "lend a hand." Lisa would also share food with them. By October, Beth's condition was worsening to the point that she now needed a wheelchair, but her spirit was never dimmed, no matter what.

In Sugar Land, adults and children in the schools, churches and neighborhood, demonstrated their care for John and Beth in so many ways. On Saturday, October 9, friends and neighbors hosted an ROTC march in conjunction with the Susan Konan Race for the Cure. The girl's high school ROTC paraded and executed their drills in John and Beth's honor in front of their houses. Pink ribbons were tied around the trees, and signs were placed in yards with well wishes spelled out for both Beth and John. Beth was brought out to the cul-de-sac to greet the parade and the neighbors. She was wearing a pink cancer awareness hat. John could no longer be transferred to his wheelchair, so his bed was placed at the best angle possible to his window, where we hoped that he could see. We told him that the marchers were there in Beth's honor and his. However, while John heard and knew, we were unable to get him or his bed in a position where he could really see much. His neck was hurting and his paralysis prevented adjusting his position in the bed so that he could view the parade. While he could hear us and understand that a parade was outside his window, he could not see it. Lisa, other family members and I went outside briefly to greet the well wishers and thank them for their efforts. They prayed with us for John and then we quickly returned to John's bedside.

During the last weeks of John's illness, his pastors Tom Pace and Jeff McDonald came often. They were present for John, praying, offering communion and whatever words of comfort and love that they could. We had our own family church services and served communion without the benefit of an ordained minister on Sundays. We were all there with him, siblings, parents, step parents, step siblings and of course most important of all, his precious Lisa, Mary Kaitlin and Carly.

Chapter 7

THE ALPHA AND OMEGA

"I love your mother, and through her, we will be connected always."

John went home to his heavenly Father on October 14, 2004. His family had been staying near his bedside all day. A new hospice nurse had come that morning to care for him as well. We were initially disappointed simply because we did not know her. But she was a God send in getting us through this terrible day. John was peaceful, mostly sleeping. His breathing was becoming shallow, he had had oxygen for about two days now, and he did not appear to be struggling to breathe. The nurse reported to us that afternoon that John was dying. She read the signs and told us what they were. Nevertheless, we did not understand, nor I'm sure did we want to understand the imminence of his death. The day wore on. I rarely left his bedside. As nighttime came, I made the decision that I would stay all night. Therefore I thought that I should make the quick 15 minute trip home to get my pajamas and toothbrush, convincing myself that John would be with us through the night. My heart and mind were still hoping for some kind of "turn-around" which would prove the nurse wrong.

About 9:00 PM, I quickly got in my car and started the 15 minute drive to my house. Almost immediately, the signal flashed on my dashboard warning me of a flat tire. I had to make a quick stop for air at the Texaco that was on my route home. After I put air in the tires, I proceeded toward my house. I realized that I was taking a little more time than I had expected to take, so I called back to check in and to explain the situation. Bob answered the phone. He said; "You had better turn around and come back right now." While waiting for my return, he asked John to hold on until Mother got there. My breaking heart was in my throat as I turned around and made my way back to my son's bedside, hoping and praying that I would not be too late.

A few minutes later, I rushed in the front door and to John's bedside. He was surrounded by his family. He was perfectly still. For an instant I was not sure – then he took a new kind of short choppy breath that had developed after I left to go home for my pajamas. "My precious son," I cried. "I love you. I love you." I touched and gently held his hand. He responded by the expression on his face and moving his head toward me. All of us knew that he recognized that his mother was there now. We prayed the Lord's Prayer and maintained our vigil with softly spoken words of love, comfort and assurance, as John continued his ever more slow and choppy breathing. Lisa told him gently how much she loved him and how much that his girls and all of us loved him. West told his brother that he did not have to worry, everything would be OK, and that he could let go now if ready. The nurse was standing by, counting seconds between his breaths. Somehow she knew to quit counting after his last breath was drawn. Then, she gently confirmed to us that it was his last.

This kind hospice nurse also knew what to do as we stood there stunned and lost. It was about 10:15 at night. Much was left to be done in accordance with laws of Texas before John's body was taken from his home after 2:00 AM. Our hospice nurse orchestrated it with skill and compassion. Remember Dr. Gustafson, the oncologist who prescribed the protocol that John followed after his first brain tumor in 1983? Dr. Gustafson was a fairly young man then. However, he had health problems in the 1990's and had closed his private practice. When we were issued John's death certificate, he was the Texas Department of Health physician who had signed it these 21 years later.

I cannot finish this story without commenting on the outpouring of love at John's death. So many had known of John's recent fight to live and many more knew of the courage with which he had overcome so much starting with his first brain tumor in 1983. Contributions flowed into the John Warren Brain Tumor Memorial Fund at the Texas A&M Health Science Center College of Medicine that Bob and I established in John's memory. Notes and letters came pouring in as well. Family and friends came from around the state to celebrate his life and mourn his death. Their support and expressions of love somehow kept us afloat. There were over 200 friends and family members who visited with us at the funeral home the night before his memorial service. Men, women and children filled the sanctuary of our large church to capacity the next day. Mary Kaitlin's entire Peer Assistance Leadership class (PALS) was excused from school to be there for her. Many of Carly's friends were there with their parents. In San Antonio, 200 friends and relatives came to the grave side to say goodbye to John. Many of them had not been able to travel to Houston for the service the day before.

At John's memorial service, our pastor Tom Pace spoke of John's kindness, patience, honesty, humility and love, saying that these attributes of John's life reflected Jesus' life. He read one of John's letters to his girls that he had written to them in August, a letter that has become so important to his children and to all of us.

Dear - my blessed children. I love you so much. The hand of Jesus is not in this disease – you are both so talented and smart. Please don't let my passing hurt your faith in the Lord. God's hand is only in good. He has brought me much comfort in these days. I am so glad you will continue.

I love your mother and through her, we will be connected always. I love you beyond measure. I am so happy that you will be living with your mother. She will need lots of love that I know you two will provide. I am so sorry I won't be there.
I will always love you both,
Daddy

Most of all I want you both to know I would never leave you.

Pastor Jeff McDonald read to the congregation a touching tribute that Mary Kaitlin had written after John's death.

<u>Mary Kaitlin Warren's Tribute to her Dad</u>

Not many people knew my dad the way I did - in fact only one other person, my sister. Dad was (it's hard to put into words) the world's greatest dad. He could crack a joke and make you smile even if you thought there would be no tomorrow. One time, I had just had my heart broken and I decided to write this guy a note. Stupid me! I left it on the table and went to softball. When I got back, the letter was completely modified. Instead of a sincere greeting, it had; "Dear Scum Bug!" Even though I was mad, I still found humor in it.

Dad, There was just something about him. If you ever read <u>Death Be Not Proud</u>, it kind of sums up how dad was. He brightened every life he touched. There was just something about him - his charm, his wit. Whatever it was, it was just really special. Those of you who were privileged as I was, to meet my Dad, know what I'm talking about.

I was always really proud of my dad. I loved to show him off to my friends in elementary school. He was like a brother and a father all in one. That sound strange but it was true. He was a kid at heart. He saw the world through the eyes of a child in my mind. He'd be like a kid on Christmas morning when he got a new pocketknife or something like that.

I came to admire his love for primitive things, like making his own bows and arrows, even if they didn't always work. His love of nature and despise of our video games - his lack of knowledge with computers. It made you really appreciate the simple things of life when you were around him. My dad had this one quote that he made up that I really like. "If you do not look, you will not see." That kind of - in my

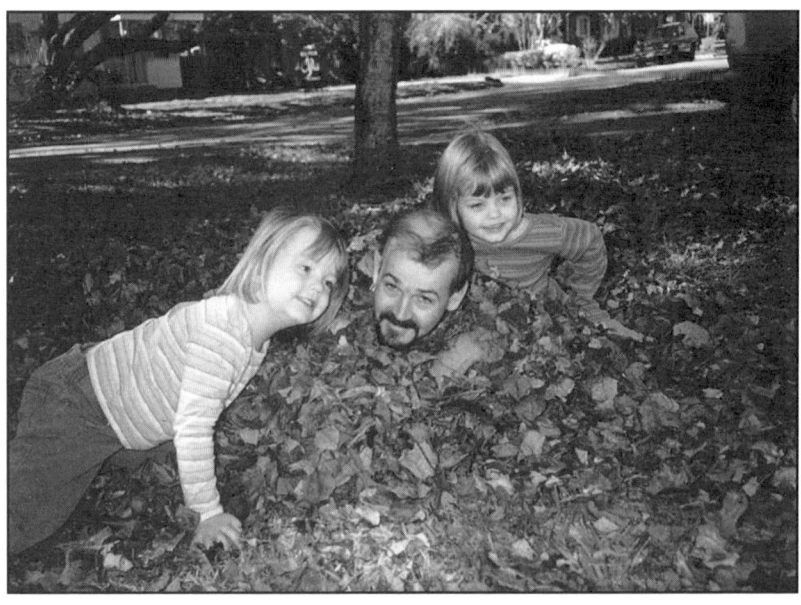

"He was a kid at heart."

opinion at least - sums up his life. Not necessarily the way he handled big things, but the way he handled ordinary things too. I don't know how to end this, so I'll just say this, my dad is definitely the Greatest Dad on Earth!

John's brother West along with his two friends, Rebe and Ashby also gave eulogies that were touching and from the heart.

<u>West's Eulogy to John</u>

As we put together the pictures you've seen today of John's life and friends and family, I could only think again of what a wonderful man he was and what an honor and blessing it has been to call him my brother. He was loyal and trustworthy- a man you could count on. He worked hard and was devoted to his family- Lisa, Mary Kaitlin, and Carly. He was kind and gentle with his children and his love for them was transparent in all that he did. His wife Lisa was his life's love- she was his angel. He was slow to anger, quick to forgive, quick to help anybody in need. He loved his friends- too many to mention all but I will mention Barbie and Reb, Ashby and Joanie, and Gary and Andrea who gave and shared with him so much love and laughter over their lives together and who were so much support to him in his final days. He loved his Mom and Dad. He loved the Lord, his church and his Pastor Tom. He loved old black and white Westerns on TV, Louis Lamour and Zane Grey novels, bows and arrows that he made from tree stumps and turkey feathers, old stuff, and old people. He talked to strangers like they were old friends and many of them became new friends. He loved his dog Bo. He found stray dogs and saw the good in them. Behind every good dog there is a good person and my brother had lots of good dogs. He saw the good in people so much more than he saw their flaws. He had not a selfish bone in his body. While his brother and buddies collected new toys to play with he did without or resurrected old stuff or made do with what he had and called it all good. He didn't covet more than the occasional pocket knife.

With stoic courage he faced the physical challenges of his disease for the last 22 years of his life. He did not surrender himself to pity or despair. Instead, he placed himself in God's hands and took each day as it came. Some days were good and some were bad, yet he was thankful for his blessings and never bitter. Most of you know the story but I'll tell it again for the record. Still in chemo 22 years ago, John got off his bed and went back to Texas A&M to earn a Petroleum Engineering Degree. Graduating just in time for the oil business to crater, he went to work in environmental consulting and remediation, first for GEO and for the past 13 years for Weston. Along the way he wore out many pairs of shoes, he found his church and his wife, and together they produced Mary Kaitlin and Carly. Lesser men could have lay down and quit and nobody would have blamed them. John got up and moved forward and never looked back. He told me more than once that if cancer had to get somebody in our family, he was glad it was him because he wouldn't want this to happen to any of us. And he meant what he said. He had great humor, rarely at anyone else's expense, but often at his own.

John loved the outdoors. He wasn't your classic hook and bullet guy- he didn't always measure his success by the game in his bag or the fish on his stringer. He loved God's creation and appreciated and respected his role in nature's never ending circle of life, death, and renewal. He loved to share his days afield or on the water with his friends and family. He was content with small pleasures. His ego consumed very little, and he was put off by those whose consumed much. He had not a pretentious bone in his body. What you saw was what you got with Brother John. He will be with me forever, in every campfire, in every gathering of family and friends, in every morning that I take to the woods, in every sunrise and sunset. He will be in my heart as I watch his children grow up into images of their father. I will hear him in our laughter and in our tears. He is the standard against which I will measure my self forever. I am honored to call him my brother. A better man I have never known.

I have learned a lot from this experience- watching my brother struggle against and suffer with this disease. I have learned that God doesn't sit at the beck and call of those who love Him, waiting in the rear like a mounted cavalry for us to direct against the enemy that causes our pain. I have learned that suffering is simply ours to bear, that we can no more eliminate it from our lives than we can eliminate the color blue from the spectrum of light. But I have also learned that in our suffering, our love for one another is perfected, and that it is in the midst of suffering that we have our clearest glimpse of what is Divine in this life. I have seen so many friends of this family who could have so easily simply retreated and insulated themselves from all of this, instead step forward and share the pain and heartbreak and suffering with John and with us. That is love, sacrificial love, the kind of love that costs you something. It is God's love for us. He is here with us, in us, around us, and among us and I have seen Him clearly in these difficult days.

For John, God was the *alpha* and *omega* and God was Love for as long as he lived on this earth. John knew he was loved, and that was the most important thing to him. His origin, his journey and his destination were defined for him by Love. He said toward the end; "I have forgotten many things, but I know that I am loved." He found meaning in his first illness because he saw from it how much he was loved. Then again, before he died, he testified in a letter to his family; "God has given me great comfort through these days." John understood God as Creator and Love. Thus John had an almost uncanny ability to experience God's presence in his life.

Rebe and Ashby, whose friendships with John date back to their middle school days and who remained with him until his death, told of the many good experiences that they had shared as they grew up together. Rebe testified to the consistency of John's kindness to others as he spoke these words; "I can honestly say that I cannot remember anything that John did against me or any of his other friends that we needed to forgive him for. John was truly a role model for those of us who have a hard time being a good person on a daily basis."

Other friends from his childhood also recalled what a kind and trustworthy friend that they had in John. The following account was given to me in a letter from Katheryn Keeton upon hearing of John's death. Katheryn was our neighbor when she and John were children. Here are her words. "John was my first friend in the circle. He was a true and loyal friend – even though he took some hits for it from the other kids. He is one of the kindest and gentlest souls I ever had the pleasure to know. His heart and light will be missed."

John's miraculous recovery from his first tumor, taught him much about what really matters in life. He learned more about the importance of caring for others. After he recovered from the first brain tumor, he occasionally was called upon by a doctor who had treated him or friends to visit with other brain tumor patients which he did to encourage them with whatever compassion and hope that he could offer. In 2003, shortly before his first surgery for the second tumor, I watched and listened as he tucked his daughters in bed for the night. He told them not to be afraid because he knew Jesus was with them in their house and everything thing would be OK. While he asked God for physical healing many times, by faith and observation, he knew that God's healing did not always come by physical healing. When he knew the end was coming, he turned to God in prayer and asked that his life be made a sacrifice, so that others in his family would never have to go through living and dying with a brain tumor. *"Let me be the lamb,"* he prayed.

And thus, from the beginning of his life to the end, John worshiped God in mind, body, spirit and for the beauty of the earth. He opened his heart and responded to God's grace with dignity and humility, and most of all by valuing loving relationships more than anything else, just as God planned for us all.

CHAPTER 8

NEW BEGINNINGS

"...and then go on with what you have been doing."

John's illness and death brought home to me how important siblings are to each other, especially how important Sally, West and John's relationships were to each other through the years together in their family of origin. They had their fair share of sibling rivalry, but also shared so much more in their day to day lives, learning from each other how to laugh, play, fight and forgive, protect, share and pull away to stake out confident claims for their own individuality. As adults, these memories of each other held them together for life. John's letters to Sally and West, written as he approached death and their response in words and deeds reveal the strength and depth of their relationships, how they have influenced and learned from each other and how they were and are forever bonded.

Sally and West had their own grieving to do, but in it they found the strength to take the first steps to lead the family as a whole back to a "new normal" as grief counselors often describe it to those freshly facing the loss of their loved one. Sally and West started the ball rolling to get us functioning again as an extended family in our supporting roles to each other and to John's beloved nuclear family, Lisa, Mary Kaitlin and Carly. John had entrusted us to take care of one another, as his letters made perfectly clear.

So as we faced our first holiday season without him, Sally and West came up with a joint plan. West would provide the place and the meat for a non-traditional Thanksgiving feast on his deer lease in the hill country southwest of San Antonio, and Sally would reschedule a trip for the extended Thanksgiving weekend that she had planned for John before his death. It was a trip to the Texas Hill country. During past holiday seasons, we would choose a time to gather together at least once for an extended family celebration. Their plan would provide different settings than our typical holiday and hopefully ease the pain of John's physical absence. Sally tells the story best in her own words.

My brother died October 14 in Houston of brain cancer, leaving behind a wife suffering from MS and grief, two young daughters, and a large extended family. After John's death, we were faced with the holidays coming too fast to do anything except hold ourselves together and weather through, still in shock from the ordeal of his illness, and not yet understanding how John's family would manage afterward.

As the oldest sister, I often take it upon myself to organize "Things We Can Do Together." For my brother's birthday gift last summer I had reserved a cabin in the Texas Hill Country on a cold, spring-fed river that I knew John and his family would enjoy, since John loved to fish, hunt, and observe all things natural. As it turned out, he was too sick to travel when the time came, and in fact too sick to go anywhere again, so I had to let the cabin go. When Thanksgiving approached, our mother begged to forgo the traditional turkey dinner (John had always carved); my surviving brother West offered to host the entire family at his deer lease for a wild game/barbeque Thanksgiving feast; I re-rented the river cabin, and we were all set for one of the two holiday hurdles. Christmas we would deal with later.

Thanksgiving Day came clear and blue, perfect for eating outdoors. A large group gathered at the lease: John's wife, Lisa; his daughters Mary Kaitlin and Carly; his siblings and our parents, step-parents, step-family, family-in-law. We ate carnivorously, just like the real Pilgrims, then hiked the hilly land to a creekside spot selected by West for the planting of three memorial pear trees, one each for John's wife and two daughters. In fact West had already planted the sapling trees, but a rise of the creek had washed them out of their beds, and they lay forlorn and bare-rooted, awaiting rescue. All hands, literally, joined in digging new holes placed a little further up the bank, the children running back and forth from the creek with 12 oz. water bottles to water the relieved pears. Afterward, we sang, swayed and held hands, accompanying West, as he played his guitar in homage to our lost husband, father, son, brother.

At the end of the peaceful day, the Hunters stayed at the lease and the Gatherers moved on, driving directly toward the setting sun, for two hours of hairpin turns over the surprisingly rough and remote Hill Country mountaintops. My husband, Jeff, blazed the trail, with my mother driving behind us in the second car, bearing the precious cargo of John's family, her speed never exceeding 20 mph. At that rate we would never get there, so we pulled her over and brokered a change of driver, hoping that Lisa might be a little more daring, especially when placed in front of us, feeling the pressure of Jeff's BMW at her back bumper. We finally arrived at the attractive cabins, eight tired Pilgrims thankful for safe passage, and checked into our assigned home for the next few days.

John and Lisa's two children and ours get along famously – most of the time – and the closeness that we felt as the four cousins drew together for comfort and support was the antidote to uncertainty and grief for all of us. The river proved to be glorious, and we all felt the sense of John being absolutely there in that beautiful place, as if the way to connect with him was to connect with what he loved: nature as Medium, clear cold water as Life, golden light as Salvation, open sky as Hope.

On the last full day, Jeff and I took the kids down to the river to a place where an old concrete bridge had washed out under the pressure of an enormous flood. The river was high from abundant rainfall, and there were modest rapids as the water flowed through the constricted passage. "Tubers" had discovered the rapids and we stood and watched an excited group float the bumpy ride. The girls and I were facing upriver as a lone figure appeared, sitting in a strangely configured fishing boat, a tall framework with a single seat, almost a paddleboat. As the fisherman drew closer, the children and I saw to our amazement the face of my brother; his sweet-natured, goateed, fishing capped countenance, eerily belonging to the stranger in the boat. John's face, perfectly calm and absorbed with his task as he positioned himself for the rough water. Then across the way, I heard Jeff's shocked voice; "Damn Sally – that looks like John." The girls and I each reached our own private conclusions and continued our talk, though our eyes lingered on the face so much like their father as he gave a friendly nod, and slipped on by us, making his way alone.

And now we, John's nuclear and extended family, were taking our first steps to make our way without him, knowing that things would never be the same, but finding our way to the "new normal" individually and collectively by supporting one another.

Chapter 9

SEARCHING

For him who has faith,
The last miracle
Shall be greater than the first.

Dag Hammarskjold, 1956

    I don't know the answers or even the questions that God would have us ask. Yet there comes a time when we must make sense of tragedy and what seems to be such unfair loss. The first time around in 1983, John experienced a modern miracle. Twenty years later, for John, the last miracle would be different than the first. This time, there would be no long term survival. Yet, I saw John's faith in action as his belief that God was with him never seemed to waver, even as he suffered and came to the realization that he was dying soon.

    John said often that he did not believe that God singled him out to have either of the two brain tumors and nor did he believe that God singled anyone out for premature death or catastrophic, tragic loss of any kind. When the tumors struck, John trusted God to do every thing that He could do in order for him to win the battles within the framework of Creation and the knowledge and resources available to his doctors. Thus, he believed that God works with and through that which he created. John trusted God to be faithful always, and in His faithfulness, John was able to see and experience God using the worst of times to bring forth goodness. For these things I am thankful.

    While I have thought and agonized over what might have been done that wasn't done for John to give him a second physical miracle, I have had to come to the conclusion that given where we are in science and medicine today, all was done that could be done within the medical community. There were medical choices to make, and by making one choice, others were excluded. Yet, I doubt that the outcome could have been much different, given the choices that were available at the time.

The truth is that 20 plus years ago John "slipped through the cracks" as one doctor said. Since then, treatment protocols for glioma brain tumors are much the same – surgery if possible, radiation and reliance on chemotherapy, even many of the same chemotherapies that were used 20 years ago. At the time of this writing, I know of no major breakthroughs that have occurred for the treatment of this most malignant form of brain tumor. Although experimental treatments hold hope for the future, the basic approach is still to "cut, burn and poison." I am not ungrateful for these drastic measures. The successes in treating many types of cancer have improved dramatically over the past twenty years because of them. Without surgery, radiation and chemotherapy, John would not have had the remarkable longevity that he did have. Yet unfortunately, for grade III and IV glioma tumors, long term survival is so rare, that it is practically non existent.

For John, twenty years after the first tumor, the surgeons could not take as much area around the new tumor as they would have liked to take, because of the its proximity to the motor strip. John's vascular system was fragile because he had had so much treatment the first time around in 1983, including the maximum dose of full brain radiation. All of the treatment that he received in the past and in the present attacked healthy as well as cancerous cells. This created even more constraints on what could be done the second time around. The chemotherapies that had seemed effective 20 years before were now more damaging to the cancer free but fragile areas of his brain and less effective in killing cancer cells.

In retrospect, I have worried that perhaps we tried too hard and encouraged John to try too hard to continue trying to extend his life. But I keep coming back to the fact that John loved life, and he passionately and courageously wanted to live in order to be with his wife and children as long as he could. He said optimistically when his second tumor was first discovered that he was hoping for another 20 years. He found out all too soon that would not happen again. Yet, after his third surgery, Dr. Prahbu asked John on two different occasions if he was glad that he had undergone that surgery. John answered affirmatively both times. The first time was while John was still in the hospital. The second time was when we had returned to his office for a follow-up visit. John was confined to his wheelchair and obviously continuing his decline. But he smiled rather sadly at the doctor and said; "I would not be here now if I had not had the surgery."

He wanted to live every day that he had gained through the procedure, and was willing to suffer more in order to have those extra days and weeks. He used those days after the final surgery to spend hours talking to Lisa about their lives and the future of Lisa and the girls. He wrote his letters that are so important for his family to have. He prayed. And he hoped against hope, trying valiantly, but with little success, to walk again as the rapidly growing cancer did not abate. And of course, John and all of his family hoped from the beginning that in giving him more time, something new would come along that would change the course of the disease.

Because glioma brain tumors are relatively infrequent in the population, they have not received as much attention as breast cancer, prostate cancer and other diseases that effect many more people every year. Even now, fewer than 4 percent of these patients survive for five years, and the fatal recurrence often occurs within the first nine months of the disease. It is one of the most lethal cancers, killing about 10,000 Americans each year, as the fast growing cells with microscopic tentacles reach as much as six inches from the visible mass destroying all healthy tissue in its wake.

More answers and more effective treatments are desperately needed. Fortunately, there is hope for this on the horizon. There are recent reports of experimental shots that are being used in clinical trials on certain cancer patients, including glioblastoma patients. Instead of poisoning the cancer, they "signal" the immune system to selectively attack the malignant cells. There is cautious optimism that immunotherapy treatments may be proven effective on some tumors without causing toxic side effects that kill healthy cells as well as malignant cells for patients like John and many others.

A front page article in the Houston Chronicle provided information on a trial that is going forward on immunotherapy. Another Chronicle article reported research on a new theory of "epigenetics" that is being conducted by a professor of Texas A&M's Institute of Biosciences and Technology in the Medical Center. According to the news report, the A&M professor is one of a growing number of scientists who say that flawed cell division causes many cancers. This theory posits that DNA letters of genes are not changed or mutated (as postulated in Genome research on genetic mutations) but that they change as a result of some other external force, like a hydrocarbon bonding with a healthy gene and stopping it from working. What is causing this to happen was reported to be "anyone's guess." But this and other lines of research should lead to a better understanding, prevention and more responsive treatments of lethal glioma brain tumors, as well as some other types of cancers.

For now, John's almost unheard of longevity after being diagnosed and treated for an Astrocytoma III in 1983 is a story of hope for other brain tumor patients. During the years that he survived to lead a normal life, he was called upon to visit with other brain tumor patients, which he did, to offer them support and hope based upon his own experience. But the best hope does not lie in "slipping through the cracks" as John did once. The best hope lies in focusing on this disease through more private and public resources being brought to bear upon research. If this happens, there should come a time when it will not be a rarity at all for one with a highly malignant brain tumor to have life extended for 20 years and beyond, as John's life was.

John often verbalized that he wanted his experience and participation in clinical trials to help others if not him. With that in mind, shortly before his death, his family established the John Warren Brain Tumor Research Fund at the College of Medicine, Texas A&M University. Approximately 175 family members and friends have made contributions to the fund. This fund, established in John's memory, will continue to grow and support faculty and students in their efforts for new and innovative research that may lead to his dream of a Plan D. The Fund is but one small pebble dropped into the larger pool of funding that is needed. But ripples from one pebble continue to spread outward providing help and encouragement in the larger pool of funding and scientific research. When in the last phase of his illness, still searching for Plan D, John looked up at me from his bed one day with a smile and said; "All things are possible."

I end the story that I have written for John by returning to Dag Hammarskjold's quote which fits John's view of life so well; *"For him who has faith, the last miracle shall be greater than the first."*

The John William Warren III Memorial Brain Tumor Fund

    The John William Warren III Memorial Brain Tumor Research Fund, Texas A&M Health Science Center College of Medicine is now providing support for the research of neuroscientist, Farida Sohrabji, Ph.D., Associate Professor of Neuroscience and Experimental Therapeutics. In the fall of 2005, Dr. Sohrabji hired the first undergraduate student as a result of this fund established in John's memory. Subsequently, the student's research focused on astrocyte cells in female rats and resulted in her placing first in the Life Sciences group during Student Research Week presentations made on the Texas A&M campus. The experience also set her on a path to her future. Beginning in the fall of 2006, she has embarked on graduate education at the University of Texas Southwestern Medical Center in order to study neuroscience. John's family is pleased with the difference John's memorial fund is already making, especially because we know that it helps to fulfill his wish that his death from a brain tumor might in someway lead to help for others. The fund is growing and the money it generates for neuroscience research is increasing.

    Proceeds from the sale of John's Story will be donated to the Memorial Brain Tumor Research Fund. Other individual contributions will be appreciated and may be made to the John William Warren Memorial Brain Tumor Fund by check payable to the HSC Foundation and mailed to the following address:

Texas A&M Health Science Center
College of Medicine
Office of Institutional Advancement
147 Joe H. Reynolds Medical Building
College Station, TX 77843-1114

Make checks payable to:
Texas A&M HSC Foundation
Memo: John Warren Fund-COM

Author's Note

I began writing my son John's memoir in January, 2005. It was important to me to write his story in my effort to cope with the terrible grief that gripped me. The story as I tell it reflects his courageous fight against a lethal brain cancer, which includes his miraculous recovery from the first tumor diagnosed in 1983. The story recounts the way that event suddenly changed his young life as a college student to the life of a determined young man who knew the odds against him, but continued to embrace living to the fullest for the next 20 years before the disease recurred in 2003. His memoirs reflect the faith, courage, humor and kindness that were his trademarks from the diagnosis and treatment of the first tumor until his death on October 14, 2004, one year and eight months after his second diagnosis.

The text is written from my memory of what transpired during those years, from poems and letters of John's that I saved, from a limited amount of my journaling and John's journaling, from suggestions and contributions from his wife Lisa, his daughters Mary Kaitlin and Carly, his brother West and Sister Sally, his father Blair and step father Bob, as well as medical records that various doctors wrote from the beginning to the end of the 21 years that John lived after his first diagnosis. Real names of people are used. There was no need to do otherwise, as all the people mentioned in his memoirs from the medical profession, to family members, friends, co-workers, neighbors and the church community contributed to his life in special and positive ways for which John was always thankful and appreciative.

My description of the County Courthouse that is across the street from the apartment John rented in Corsicana came from <u>The Courthouses of Texas</u>, a guide by Mavis P. Kelsey, Sr., and Donald H. Dyal, published by the Texas A&M University Press.

When writing about trees that John loved, I found additional information about the "bodark" tree from a book intitled <u>Forest Trees of Texas</u>, published by the Texas Forest Service, a part of The Texas A&M University System.

I cite two reports on current cancer research from articles that I found in the Houston Chronicle in 2006. Both are cited as examples of current research efforts that may offer hope for brain tumor patients in the future.

In closing John's memoir, I used a fitting quote from Dag Hammarskjold that was cited in a book that I was reading at the time entitled <u>Streams of Living Water</u> by Richard J. Foster, page 260. Foster's source was Hammarshkjold's book <u>Markings</u>, page 172.

A brief sketch of author's life

I was born in Waco, TX on January 1, 1936. I was married to Frank Blair Warren in 1955. I have three children by my first marriage, Sally, West and John Warren. John was the youngest of the three. I have been married to Robert "Bob" Elliott White, MD, a psychiatrist, since 1978. Our blended family includes my three children and his three children, Rene, Scott, and Kim. All of our children are grown and we are a very close and "well blended" family. We have 8 grandchildren, ranging in ages from 4 to 21 years of age. After my three children were in grade school or above, I went back to school in San Antonio, receiving a BA degree in 1970 from the University of Incarnate Word, and an MS in Urban Studies from Trinity University in San Antonio in 1972. I worked in the Planning Department of the City of San Antonio from 1972 until 1978, when I married Bob. Then I moved to the Houston area, where I worked as the City Planner for the City of Bellaire for 10 years. In 1988, I decided to leave Bellaire to pursue a Ph.D. at Rice University in political science with a focus on state and local government. I received my Ph.D. from Rice in 1994. After leaving my staff position in Bellaire, I continued as a planning consultant in Bellaire and other small towns and major cities in the region. During my career, I have been active in the American Planning Association, holding leadership positions at the national, state and local levels, including a term as the Texas State Chapter President. I am a member of the American Institute of Certified Planners and was inducted into their College of Fellows in 2000. I am now retired, and spending my time with family, especially John's wife and two daughters who live in Sugar Land near Bob and me.

Sara Jane White, Ph.D., FAICP